# Qigong
# for Living

A Practical Guide for Improving Your Health
with Qi from Modern China

BY YANLING LEE JOHNSON

**YMAA Publication Center**
**Boston, Mass. USA**

**YMAA Publication Center**
Main Office:
4354 Washington Street
Boston, Massachusetts, 02131
617-323-7215 • ymaa@aol.com • www.ymaa.com

POD1008

ISBN:1-886969-11-6

Edited by Susan Bullowa
Cover design by Katya Popova

**Publisher's Cataloging in Publication**
*(Prepared by Quality Books Inc.)*

Johnson, Yanling Lee.
   Qigong for living : a practical guide for improving
your health with qi from modern China / by Yanling Lee
Johnson. — 1nd ed.
      p. cm.
   Includes bibliographical references and index.
   LCCN: 20028595
   ISBN: 1-886969-11-6

   1. Qi gong.  2. Physical fitness. 3. Health.
I. Title.

RA781.8.J64 2002          613.7'1
                          QBI33-593

**Disclaimer:**
   The authors and publisher of this material are NOT RESPONSIBLE
in any manner whatsoever for any injury which may occur through reading
or following the instructions in this manual.
   The activities, physical or otherwise, described in this material may be
too strenuous or dangerous for some people, and the reader(s) should
consult a physician before engaging in them.

Printed in USA.

# Table of Contents

**Foreword** . . . . . . . . . . . . . . . . . . . . . . . . . . . . . . . . . . . . . . . . . .**v**

**Preface** . . . . . . . . . . . . . . . . . . . . . . . . . . . . . . . . . . . . . . . . . . . .**vi**

**Dedication & Acknowledgments** . . . . . . . . . . . . . . . . . . . . . . . . .**xiii**

**Chapter 1. Qigong, Soul, and Spirit** . . . . . . . . . . . . . . . . . . . . . . . .**1**

Introduction . . . . . . . . . . . . . . . . . . . . . . . . . . . . . . . . . . . . . . . .1
Qigong . . . . . . . . . . . . . . . . . . . . . . . . . . . . . . . . . . . . . . . . . . .2
Soul . . . . . . . . . . . . . . . . . . . . . . . . . . . . . . . . . . . . . . . . . . . . .8
Spirit–Shen . . . . . . . . . . . . . . . . . . . . . . . . . . . . . . . . . . . . . .15

**Chapter 2. Dao and the Practice of Qigong** . . . . . . . . . . . . . . . . . .**18**

Daoism and Qigong . . . . . . . . . . . . . . . . . . . . . . . . . . . . . . . .18
Qigong Practice and the Ways of Thought in the East . . . . . . . . . . . . . .19
Sources of Daoism . . . . . . . . . . . . . . . . . . . . . . . . . . . . . . . . .20
I Ching and Qigong . . . . . . . . . . . . . . . . . . . . . . . . . . . . . . . . .21
Defining the Dao in the I Ching . . . . . . . . . . . . . . . . . . . . . . . . . .22

**Chapter 3. Qigong and Modern Investigations** . . . . . . . . . . . . . . . .**26**

Qi Energy is Unlike Any Energy We Know . . . . . . . . . . . . . . . . . .27
Qigong Healing Compared with Western Medicine . . . . . . . . . . . . . .29
What Can Qi Do? . . . . . . . . . . . . . . . . . . . . . . . . . . . . . . . . . .33
What is Qi? . . . . . . . . . . . . . . . . . . . . . . . . . . . . . . . . . . . . . .35

**Chapter 4. Immortality** . . . . . . . . . . . . . . . . . . . . . . . . . . . . . . . . .**36**

Defining Immortality in Chinese . . . . . . . . . . . . . . . . . . . . . . . .36
Practice of Immortality and the Human Body . . . . . . . . . . . . . . . . .37
Practice of Immortality as a Human Science . . . . . . . . . . . . . . . . . .38
Shen Tong in Immortality Practice . . . . . . . . . . . . . . . . . . . . . . . .38
Guidance from Spirit Teachers . . . . . . . . . . . . . . . . . . . . . . . . . .39
Spirit Types . . . . . . . . . . . . . . . . . . . . . . . . . . . . . . . . . . . . . .41
Types of Immortals . . . . . . . . . . . . . . . . . . . . . . . . . . . . . . . . .45
Achieving the Celestial and Buddha Levels . . . . . . . . . . . . . . . . . .46
Immortality Practice in Chinese and Tibetan Buddhism . . . . . . . . . . . .47
The Eight Immortals . . . . . . . . . . . . . . . . . . . . . . . . . . . . . . . .49

**Chapter 5. Qi and Life** . . . . . . . . . . . . . . . . . . . . . . . . . . . . . . . . . .**62**

How Qi and the Physical Body are Related . . . . . . . . . . . . . . . . . .62
How Our Physical Body and Soul/Spirit are Related . . . . . . . . . . . . .65
Intuition . . . . . . . . . . . . . . . . . . . . . . . . . . . . . . . . . . . . . . . .67
How the Inner Being is Revealed . . . . . . . . . . . . . . . . . . . . . . . .70

**Chapter 6. Qigong Phenomena** . . . . . . . . . . . . . . . . . . . . . . . . . . .**76**

Introduction . . . . . . . . . . . . . . . . . . . . . . . . . . . . . . . . . . . . . .76

Manifestations of Qi Power . . . . . . . . . . . . . . . . . . . . . . . . . . . . . . . . . . . . .79
What is Pi Gu . . . . . . . . . . . . . . . . . . . . . . . . . . . . . . . . . . . . . . . . . . . . . . . .87
Human Aura . . . . . . . . . . . . . . . . . . . . . . . . . . . . . . . . . . . . . . . . . . . . . . . . .93
Rainbow Lights . . . . . . . . . . . . . . . . . . . . . . . . . . . . . . . . . . . . . . . . . . . . . . .94
Natural Mummies . . . . . . . . . . . . . . . . . . . . . . . . . . . . . . . . . . . . . . . . . . . . .95

**Chapter 7. Qigong and Sexual Relationships** . . . . . . . . . . . . . . . . . . . . .**99**
The Inferior Status of Women in Chinese Culture . . . . . . . . . . . . . . . . . . . .99
Defining Sex in Chinese . . . . . . . . . . . . . . . . . . . . . . . . . . . . . . . . . . . . . .103
Qigong and the Sexual Lives of Couples . . . . . . . . . . . . . . . . . . . . . . . . . .105
The Split into the Northern and Southern Daoist Schools . . . . . . . . . . . . . .108
Practical Advice about Sexual Practices . . . . . . . . . . . . . . . . . . . . . . . . . . .114
Concerns About Qigong Practice and Sex . . . . . . . . . . . . . . . . . . . . . . . . .118
Bedroom Skills for Prolonging Healthy Lives . . . . . . . . . . . . . . . . . . . . . . .121

**Chapter 8. Qigong Exercises and Refining Qi** . . . . . . . . . . . . . . . . . . .**124**
Preparation . . . . . . . . . . . . . . . . . . . . . . . . . . . . . . . . . . . . . . . . . . . . . . .124
Practicing the Forms . . . . . . . . . . . . . . . . . . . . . . . . . . . . . . . . . . . . . . . .129
Meditation . . . . . . . . . . . . . . . . . . . . . . . . . . . . . . . . . . . . . . . . . . . . . . . .133

**Chapter 9. The Healing Power of Qigong and Modern Chinese
Medicine** . . . . . . . . . . . . . . . . . . . . . . . . . . . . . . . . . . . . . . . . . .**140**
Qigong Practice and Modern Experiments . . . . . . . . . . . . . . . . . . . . . . . . .142
Qigong—Healing Illnesses . . . . . . . . . . . . . . . . . . . . . . . . . . . . . . . . . . . .146
Medical Investigations on Qigong Treatments . . . . . . . . . . . . . . . . . . . . . .159
Translation from Master Ou Wen-Wei's Work . . . . . . . . . . . . . . . . . . . . . . .165

**Glossary** . . . . . . . . . . . . . . . . . . . . . . . . . . . . . . . . . . . . . . . . . . . . . . . . .**168**

**References** . . . . . . . . . . . . . . . . . . . . . . . . . . . . . . . . . . . . . . . . . . . . . . . .**171**

**About the Author** . . . . . . . . . . . . . . . . . . . . . . . . . . . . . . . . . . . . . . . . . . .**175**

**Index** . . . . . . . . . . . . . . . . . . . . . . . . . . . . . . . . . . . . . . . . . . . . . . . . . . . .**176**

## Foreword

Qigong practice awakens and develops our energy system. Our energy system is a complete system with a structure and complexity equal to our physical systems. Qigong is a refined science. Through personal practice, we can harness and direct energy, and gain an understanding of energy—our own energy configurations and those of others. Then, we are no longer limited by the boundaries of the material world. In other words, we are able to go beyond the boundaries of this world that seem to limit us.

Qigong is suitable for people of all ages and all physical conditions, and helps heal those who are seriously ill from conditions such as cancer, diabetes, paralysis, asthma, kidney diseases, and cardiovascular diseases.

Through qigong practice, we can combine body and soul to heal; separate body and soul to understand. Yanling details many of the finer nuances of qigong practice in her book. She brings into modern life what this powerful ancient system offers.

Mingtang Xu

Lineage Holder of ZY Qigong

## Preface

I believe qigong will blossom in this beautiful, spiritual land of America.

I am experimenting with my life, trying to climb the "mountain" of human myth and share with you what I have learned. I started writing and translating three books at the same time on qigong and herbal foods in 1993, finished *Qi, The Treasure and Power of Your Body* in 1996 in a hurry, hoping to meet the increasing qigong beginners' needs. At the same time, when I found that this Giant American "Toddler" (talking about not just eating well, but eating right) needed to know about foods, I began to focus on translating *Herbal Food For Longevity and Vitality* because Chinese has a 5,000-year-old history of eating right and is a "gold mine" of diets. This partial translation—but already a 1,500 page-book—is from one of the most important ancient Chinese medical books that supplies a complete picture of foods used for healing and longevity. I finished it in spring 1997 and then began writing this book, *Qigong Phenomena*, and finished it in the same year in September. But the first book that has been published by the YMAA Publication Center is my "youngest baby" – my fifth book that I started in 1998, *A Woman's Qigong Guide*. Finally, my *Qigong for Living* is reaching my readers.

When I am writing, I always keep in mind the ancient Chinese teaching, "Do not leave a legacy of trouble. A bad teaching can be a crime." I write not to become well known, but to build a stepping stone for those of who plan to study qigong and give you a more than just a glimpse into the world of mystical human potentials. My goal is to bring some information to English speakers who want to explore Dao. I also want my readers to understand how research differs between the East and West. Remember that many ancient sages' experiences reflect the characteristics and the needs of their times even while the sages themselves are timeless.*

Before you begin reading about qigong, I would like to give you a general background of qigong in modern China as well as a bit of its ancient history. Here I want to focus more on recent developments especially on people who are involved in medical practice.

In the thirties, newspapers in China reported a debate between Western medicine doctors and qigong masters about whether qi (pronounced "chi") could kill viruses and germs or not. According to a letter in the *Qigong & Science* magazine (4, 1994), journalists at that time wrote about Master Situ Qi's challenge to the Shanghai hospital and the government's health department. He claimed he could settle the debate by volunteering himself for experiments that combined qigong with science. He offered to be exposed to the most acute viruses that the hospital found difficult to treat, such as tuberculosis, smallpox, typhoid, cholera, and scrofula, and yet would not be infected. The government, the medical scientific and research institutes, and the hospitals all refused to consider what he had to say and did not allow him to volunteer.

After Mao Zedong took power in mainland China in 1949, he began suppressing qigong masters and religions, forcing many qigong masters to hide their identities for many years. Enduring one attack after another, many types of qigong "disappeared" from the public or emigrated from China. Due to the humble, compromising Daoist nature of qigong, many high-level qigong masters never allowed themselves to reveal their powers during most of their lifetime.

In 1970, a pioneering qigong master who was also a professor at the Beijing Artistic Institute, Guo Lin organized a group to practice qigong openly in the parks. Grand Master Guo voluntarily taught groups ranging from one to ten students. In time, more people began joining her classes that taught her qigong style, Guo Lin New Qigong Treatments. Now she has tens of thousands of students, including those from all over the world.

As soon as the government policy became more open when Deng Xiao-Ping took power in 1976, several pioneers began to promote qigong. The extrasensory abilities demonstrated by qigong practitioners took time for the general public to understand, including scientists and some government leaders. It took an open-minded senior leader, General Zhang Zhen-Huan, to stand up and give full support to the qigong masters. Zhang was the former head of the Central Science and Technology Commission of the Chinese Defense

---

*In this book, I use the term Dao instead of the more widely known term, Tao. Dao (pronounced "Dow") reflects its actual pronunciation in Chinese. I also use the term Daoism for the same reason.

Department and one of the main leaders of the Chinese space and atomic bomb experiments. After retiring, he devoted himself to qigong research and study, and encouraged qigong masters help the public.

To promote qigong, General Zhang wanted to convince people of the value of qigong by establishing scientific evidence from laboratory results. He took a group of advanced qigong masters to travel around the country. He repeatedly tested the masters in laboratories and also personally reviewed articles written by journalists about the experiments to verify their accuracy. He made sure that the reportage faithfully reflected what happened during the demonstrations and experiments. He alerted the journalists and scientists to distinguish skills gained from practice and extrasensory abilities present in the masters. He especially warned the public about qigong frauds, that is, the false masters who took advantage of people's beliefs in qigong and qigong's increasing popularity.

In 1978, after Guo Lin Qigong had already became popular, the Soaring Crane Qigong originated by Grand Master Zhao Jin-Xiang form appeared in the public and quickly won over many people far and wide. Master Zhao had been so sickly that he had to retire in his thirties. A qigong master taught Zhao qigong. After Zhao cured himself of his multiple illnesses by practicing qigong, he began to teach people in the parks. At that time, many people had become sick during the ten-year Cultural Revolution. More and more people practiced Soaring Crane because this qigong form improved their health and helped them regain their strength. Some of Zhao's students were thrown into jail because the police accused them of playing witchcraft. At that time, qigong theory had not been well explained to the public. People did not understand the spontaneous movements that occurred during an advanced practice, the Standing Meditation. The different causes of illnesses meant that people's movements were different and some even seemed as if they were acting crazy—even to the point of laughing or crying. Over twenty million people who persistently practice Soaring Crane Qigong have improved their health and have been healed of many illnesses. The Chinese government found that qigong helped them save large sums of money. Ever since the first publicly and widely practiced qigong forms, such as the Wild Goose and the Soaring Crane, were introduced in China after the late

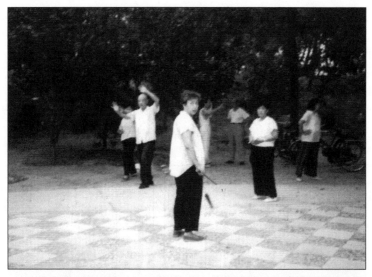

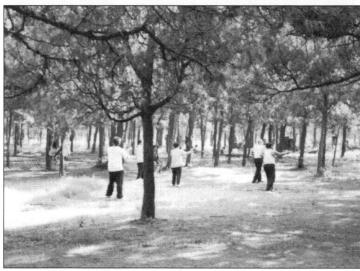

*Morning Qigong practice in a park in Beijing.*

1970s, a few thousand types of qigong have appeared. Now, qigong has become a popular movement in China.

In 1979, Chen Bin-Kui, the head of the Traditional Chinese Medicine Bureau hosted the First Qigong and Science Conference. Reports on treating cancer and the amazing qigong demonstrations convinced the attending government leaders to promote qigong. In the same year, the magazine, *Qigong & Science* was first published.

In 1984, the first Qigong Research Academic Institute was established in Beijing. Several researchers such as Dr. Grand Master Chen Fu-Yin have persevered in maintaining their research work. Following suit, the National Aeronautical Department, the National Athletic Council, and the Central Propaganda Department all issued permission for founding local qigong research academic institutes, thus prompting many provincial congresses to show support for qigong. Since the 1980s, similar institutes have been established in all provinces except Tibet and Taiwan. Also more extensive experiments were carried out in hospitals, universities, and in scientific and research institutes. Qigong is also used in military experiments and in training soldiers. Because of highly placed leaders like General Zhang Zhen-Huan, Dr. Feng Li-Da, and others, qigong has been given opportunities to show evidence of its power in scientific laboratories. These extensive experiments have proven to the world that qi is real. Some of these experiments are described later in this book.

Since 1988, more and more great qigong masters who have amazing extrasensory abilities come out of hiding. To name a few, Tian Rei-Shen, young masters like Ji Lian-Yuan, Fan Tian-Lian, Wang Yiu-Cheng, Shen Chang, Liu Xin-Yu, Sun Chu-Lin, Chen Lin-Feng, Yu Qi, Wang Bin and Wang Qiang, Wei Tian-Po, Huang Rin-Tian, Liang Guang-Xiang, and Colonel Fu Song-Shan. They all have demonstrated their abilities in front of hundreds of thousands of people and government leaders. There have been many more who have helped others in secret such as the teachers of the young masters. These teachers could very well be a garbage man who looks sloppy; a fisherman who reeks of fish; someone who walks on the street; or a monk or a Daoist who rarely meet people.

In 1988, the Chinese Federal Education Department asked Wu Han University to establish a Qigong Teacher Program to train teachers for other universities in China. Forty percent of the students in the first class in the program were selected, including some professors who did not believe in qigong. Interestingly, of those who did not believe in qigong, all developed greater extrasensory abilities by the time the class was ended, whereas only half of all students gained extrasensory abilities.

Newly established qigong schools and the more open environment has produced many qigong healers such as Mr. Jiang Chang-

Wen, the retired chairman of the Meteorological Bureau of Hunan Province, who devotes himself to treating patients for free. His motivation came from his own experience. Before he was involved in qigong, Jiang had been hospitalized several times and stayed in the hospital for a number of years without becoming well. He had acute hepatitis, nephritis, high blood pressure, gallstones, and heart disease. He was so weak that he sometimes fainted. After a serious operation, his digestion became even worse. At that time, a good friend told him about qigong which he then tried. After he learned and practiced diligently, his health improved. By the time he turned 70 years old in 1995, he was in not only in excellent condition, but was also a well-known qigong healer. He has treated many diseases and is especially successful in treating "stone" cases. On the shelves in his clinic, there are 628 small bottles that contain stones that he has removed from his patients' organs, such as kidneys and gall bladders. No medicine and no operation was ever needed, just his qigong treatment. He continues to help people, and tells them how qigong has saved his life and enables him to help others.

On January 30, 1994, at the National Qigong Conference, General Zhang gave his farewell speech. He encouraged qigong practitioners and professionals to continue their scientific experiments and research for the benefit of the people. He said that qigong masters shoulder a heavy responsibility for mankind. Three months later, he died peacefully at the age of seventy-nine. Despite the loss of this champion of qigong who supported qigong masters and research with as much devotion and power, qigong still spreads quickly in China as soon as it gets the chance. The Chinese people have been convinced since ancient times that everyone has the inner power—qi—for healing, vitality, and longevity. When I visited Beijing in June 1999, I saw many more people practicing qigong at the gates of the parks and in the streets during the early morning hours than I had seen in 1987.

Today, more and more well-respected institutes support qigong. Hospitals are finding its true value repeatedly in qigong laboratory experiments with qigong masters. Some scientists have even been alarmed by their results because they could not explain to other scientists elsewhere what had happened and how qigong was able to change the nature of some materials previously thought and proven to be unchangeable. Some of the results have been kept secret. The qigong phenomena displayed by qigong masters have recurred many times under experimental conditions, even those done without instrumentation. Feats that are ordinarily done only with sophisticated instruments were accomplished with the bare hands of these masters. The experimental evidence has convinced many well-known Chinese scientists, scholars, and many influential people who are not used believing phenomena without a scientific base. In this book, I describe some of the laboratory evidence and clinical research.

By 1997, more than a hundred grand qigong masters left China. Their reasons varied: lack of support from the government and weariness with the endless requests from the senior government leaders for treatments were often cited. Rumors had it that seven qigong masters were requested to give Deng Xiao-Ping qi treatment each day. Some masters were troubled by the daily hundreds of thousands of visitations by those who sought help. Qigong in China, however, is developing rapidly year after year despite the political situation. There is hope that the wishes of the pioneers such as Master Situ will come true: qigong and science will become one field to serve the world.

Although disrupted by political events, Chinese media contributes much to the promotion of qigong in newspapers and qigong magazines, news reports on qigong appear daily, much like news about drug advances in the United States. The Guang Ming Newspaper, a nationally distributed paper, often sends journalists to follow qigong experiments in several hospitals. Their reportage on qigong helped the general populace explore ways to improve and stabilize their health much in the way newspapers in the United States give general advice and descriptions about diet and exercise.

## Dedication & Acknowledgments

I dedicate this book to the many qigong masters, doctors, and researchers as well as to the patients who have done noteworthy experiments that have made great, incredible contributions to medical science. I dedicate this book to the great Daoist master, late Chairman of the National Daoist Religion in China, Chen Ying-Ning and to Dr. Feng Li-Da who has engaged in a most meaningful, most important research that will benefit mankind.

My acknowledgments to my editor Susan Bullowa and to the director of the YMAA Publication Center, David Ripianzi who has never hesitated to help me.

# CHAPTER 1

# Qigong, Soul, and Spirit

## Introduction

My purpose in writing this book is to share with you some extraordinary information about human life—the phenomena of qigong in the lives of real people. You can take what I write as entertainment or use the information to learn about Chinese culture. For people who are seeking a safe way to heal, stay healthy, and prolong life, there is no doubt in my mind that qigong is the best way. For people who are interested in digging into the roots of being human, this information can help with their explorations. For people who seek more, such as spiritual enlightenment, the truth is that qigong can be simple and it can also be a difficult, long journey depending on one's goals. The ancient sages explored many paths of achieving the more advanced human evolution. To pursue the higher goals requires much effort and hard work, especially when achieving self-confidence and wisdom. This is why immortals or celestials, those who have achieved these goals, are still a minority among us.

The concepts of soul, spirit, and ghost as well as heaven and hell appeared in all cultures in the world long before the different cultures knew about each other. Was this simply because of the ancient people's fears about the phenomena and happenings that they did not understand? Were those phenomena true or not? To find out more about these concepts, I have been studying and researching classic Chinese books and sources from other cultures, learning from different grand qigong masters who have certain control of their soul/spirits, and also learning from my own qigong practice. My personal experiences have not proven all that the ancient sages handed down, but they have proven some things to me of what the sages described about the human body. I am writing this chapter as much for myself so we can discuss and probe the truth of life together. I want to share with you my culture—formed from a blend of Daoism, Buddhism, and Confucianism—that has been experimenting with qi, life, and spirit for thousands of years.

Many people are searching for the truth of life, including scientists. Some are trying to find out why and how we human beings are able to think and feel, and whether having such abilities exist because we have brains and nerve systems. Modern science has carried out many genetic experiments, discovered DNA, and succeeded in cloning animals. No one is sure, however, about the soul and spirit that many people have experienced in their lives, including hundreds of thousands of qigong practitioners. That a soul and a life are directly related is the same belief in all cultures. Some differences in these beliefs, as well as the theory how a life starts, exist between Chinese culture and the rest of the world.

## Qigong

DEFINING QIGONG

Qi—gong are two words in the Chinese language that are directly related to each other. Qi is pronounced "chi". *Qi* means energy (or vitality) and *gong* means practice and cultivation. Qigong, which originated from the ancient philosophy of qi in Daoism, includes tools that can help people to become free of the need for health care. Qigong practice and cultivation can help practitioners take charge of their own physical health and mental balance. They are practices designed to strengthen the ability to absorb qi and purify qi, an ability that humans are born with and which has often become polluted. There are many stories in China about real people whose qigong practice has helped them become healthier, more confident about themselves, nicer, wiser, more intelligent, more forgiving, more optimistic, even less jealous, less wildly arrogant, and more philosophical. Qigong can function in all of the following ways:

> *Qigong can ideally adjust and improve one's entire nervous system.*
> *Qigong can improve blood circulation, breathing system, and internal organs.*

*Qigong can change and improve the muscles, bones, and tendons.*

*Qigong can strengthen immunity.*

*Qigong can improve the digestive system.*

*Qigong can ideally adjust the temperature of the body and the skin.*

*Qigong can remove or give off energy through exercise, and that energy can even change the shape or nature of some living things.*

*Qigong is an individual scientific experiment and is a life science experiment.*

There is so much that qigong can do. Human beings have used qigong over a very long time for healing and prolonging life. Knowing more about how long qigong has been practiced on our planet can help you understand not only how Chinese culture developed into a qi-based culture, but also about the benefits of learning qigong. So please follow me in tracing the root of qigong.

## THE ANCIENT HISTORY OF QIGONG

Since ancient times, qigong is the way the Chinese ancestors taught people to follow nature in preserving health, achieving longevity, and more. Looking at how the Chinese characters are written can show the relationships. For example, the word for sky, heaven is tian. Tian (天)is formed by two other characters, human (ren) (人) and two (二). Interestingly, when you make the top stroke of tian tilted like this, (夭), a totally different word that means dead, yao, is formed. But when you make the stroke for the word human sticking out of the two lines that means two, another character meaning man, fu (夫) is formed. The different means of changing the way heaven (tian) is written hints at qigong theory; that is, when you follow the natural law, you remain alive; when the natural law is not carried in the "straight" way, you will be dead. When you move beyond the natural law in the qigong way, you become a "real man." This theory is described in further detail in the chapter about immortality.

Grand Qigong Master and Traditional Chinese Medicine (TCM) physician Yan Xin said that an item unearthed from Gan Su province in China further proved that qigong has had a very long history. This

5,000-year-old clay jar found in west China in 1975 has a painting of a person who was practicing qigong; the figure has a man's head, but a woman's body. The formal, officially written Chinese record about qigong in Chinese history is at least 3,700 years old. At that time, many more books were written about qigong practices; some of these authors are unknown. Later, the religions of Daoism and Buddhism were established (2,300 years ago). Qigong also developed in the Daoist and Buddhist monasteries, as well as in the practice of Confucianism and among the people. While the separate groups formed their own styles, they relate to one another in an integrated way and all approach the highest level in the same way. Even today, nobody is 100% percent sure exactly how long qigong has been practiced on our planet. Daoism, Buddhism, and Confucianism were all established at least a couple of thousands later. There is more information in my *A Woman's Qigong Guide* about this topic. In the following paragraphs, I'll introduce you to some ancient qigong masters.

In Chinese mythology, a man by the name of Pan Gu was said to grow out of qi, and then "created the universe, and created all living things from qi." In my research on Daoism, I found that all deities in Chinese mythology were in charge of qi that affect our beings in different ways, such as the qi in white color that affects the lung; yellow that affects the spleen/stomach; or green that affects the liver. A skilled Traditional Chinese Medicine doctor can diagnose diseases from areas of darkness in the patients' facial aura. A qigong master with an opened third eye can see the colors of the human aura; a blue color would indicate that the person was having positive thoughts at the time.

The first Chinese Emperor-Sage, Shen Nong had a teacher who was a grand qigong master. Shen Nong revealed an ability to scan (that is, see something with the third eye) things such as his own internal organs. He used this ability to look for useful herbs and tested them on himself. He then observed how they affected his organs and how the herb worked inside his body first before he began teaching his people.

The Yellow Emperor himself was a great qigong master and physician. His own great teacher, Peng Zu, was said to have lived for at least 400 years (in some other books, it said that he lived about

1,200 years.). Peng Zu taught the Yellow Emperor how people should dwell in harmony with natural laws and how to use remedies for attaining ripe old age. He found that people who lived on qi lived longer than people who lived on grains.

A book, *Guan Zi* (which also the author's name) written sometime between 475–221 BC included many articles that describe in detail about qigong masters who explored their extrasensory abilities. Guan Zi explained in his book how universal qi exists, exchanges, and moves; how qi from the universe mingles with the lives on the earth; and how qi can reveal a person's extrasensory abilities. He expressed these ideas in a metaphor that "a human's body is like a house; if it is clean, then the guest, that is, the qi from the universe, would like to come and visit." The word, qi was used in other books that preceded his book, such as the *I Ching* and *Dao De Jing*. Note that the character for *jing* in the title of *The Yellow Emperor Essential Internal Jing* and in many other ancient books is the same word as it is in the book, Yin Fu Jing. This jing is a different character from the jing in jing, qi, and shen. The first jing character means "classic, important books." It can also mean "path"—a path that the ancient sages used to guide people.

Another book, *Zhou Yi Tsan Tong Qi* written during the period between 25-220 AD by a great Daoist immortal, Wei Bo-Yang, describes the universe. The book says that the primeval state of the universe was chaos full of matter and motion of qi, and goes on to describe how qi produced lives and how, in the natural world, living things are connected to qi. The author explained how practicing qigong helps people adapt to nature. The book described how the movement of the stars affects us and how a qigong practitioner benefits from using the position of Big Dipper and its handle in their practice. In many historical records as well as in almost all the classic novels, qigong masters' performances of their extrasensory abilities are described vividly. Books like these have nourished the Chinese culture and medicine as well as qigong.

Qigong has endured and has become strong today primarily because of its healing power, vitality, and potentials and also because it does not have rigid, overly elaborated rules. For example, a student could become his teacher's teacher if the student achieved a higher level than his teacher. One such story is about Immortal Xu Xun who is famous because his whole family flew physically in front of the public. Immortal Xu learned from Immortal Wu Meng, and then met a higher level teacher named Immortal Chen Mu. Immortal Xu mastered all what Immortal Chen Mu taught him, including making herbal formulas for speeding up the practice of immortality. Immortal Chen Mu told Immortal Wu to study from Xu, and Wu became Xu's student.

Qigong theory is the foundation of Chinese herbal medicine and diet that considers prevention its first priority; this is accomplished by balancing qi in harmony with the body. In order to harmonize the qi in the patient's whole system, an experienced Traditional Chinese Medicine (TCM) doctor listens to the patient's voice; checks the facial color; and feels the pulse to check the qi movements. He may also smell the patient's breath, look at his tongue, or check the stool to diagnose the disease. The doctor looks at the patient as a whole being just as qigong works on the whole body. The ancient Daoist grand masters emphasized that before learning Dao, one should learn some Chinese medicine because health and Daoism are closely related. In my *A Woman's Qigong Guide,* I explained this concept in more detail.

Most ancient books written in Chinese about qigong by well-known grand qigong masters of Daoism and Buddhism described the different spiritual dimensions. A person's soul can choose either to stay on the earth in physical or in spiritual form, or to travel to look for a better house (that is, another body) to occupy. Another choice is to continue her practice in order to become a higher level being such as an immortal celestial.

Chinese qigong has endured also because it has absorbed nourishment from other cultures such as Buddhism that originally came from India. Because of its shared essential philosophy with Daoism, the Chinese people readily accepted Buddhism two thousand years ago. A master monk from India by the name of Boddhidharma (referred to by the Chinese as Potidarmo) (around 520 AD) created the Buddhist chan (zen in Japanese), another style of qigong practice. The Chinese people call him the Chan-Ancestor Da Mo. Potidarmo was the 28th successor of the Lord Buddha who planted the root of Chan practice in China that later spread to Japan.

Further demonstrating the tolerant nature of Daoism, China was the only country to have accepted some Jewish people to settle down and live in harmony more than one thousand years ago. A Jewish synagogue still exists in Quan Zhou City in the Fujian province.

Because qiqong easily melds with other cultural influences, it has developed into approximately five thousand forms, according to the research of Dr. Liu Tian-Jun. Qigong is still a self-effort practice, no matter if it takes place under a religious name or not. You can see that qigong should be not confused with a religion although there are many qigong practices that come under religious mantles such as Daoism or Buddhism.

QIGONG AS A SELF-EFFORT PRACTICE

The Chinese Yellow Emperor (about 5,000 years ago) warned qigong masters not to teach superstitious people because only by not being superstitious, are people able to learn more about themselves from qigong practice. Not only the Yellow Emperor, but also the sages whom people called Buddha, Daoist deities, and celestials told their students repeatedly that they themselves were only human beings who explored their human potential to a higher degree. Lao Zi, the author of *Dao De Jing*, was a grand qigong master and a philosopher; the Lord Buddha himself was a grand qigong master, a healer, and a philosopher; Confucius was a philosopher and a qigong master. From what I have studied about Jesus, I think he was also a great qigong master, healer, and philosopher. He told his disciples. "If you want to know who I am, you must first know yourself." All these sages emphasized "self-effort" including the great sage, Jesus. Only not being superstitious can a practitioner work on gaining the ultimate attainment of human beings. Possibly, we will live and not die in the way that the sages said about many people, "They die muddleheaded without knowing the truth of life."

Qigong practice is a human science, yet one that can only be proven by self-cultivation. Without putting forth what is called "self-effort" and lacking experience, qigong practitioners cannot bring themselves close to their own inner being, and as a result can be fooled by false masters. Some qigong masters are deluded and think of themselves as gods after they have explored some human potential. They tell their students that they can induce their gong even when the students are not practicing. There are also some fraudulent masters who take advantage of weak-minded women who think they are receiving help, but are used only to satisfy the "masters" sexually. This is why you must always use your own wisdom, and to study in order to become knowledgeable.

The self-effort also includes healing illnesses. Yes, a good qigong master or healer can give the patient a "push" up the "hill" of healing. Without coordinated self-effort practice, it is not easy to get rid of disease. When a patient has some qigong knowledge, she can cooperate with the healer while not totally and blindly depending on the healer. An experienced qigong practitioner can usually tell when a healer or teacher is unqualified although they bear qigong titles, lecture on so-called "Buddhism" and "Daoism", or perform hocus-pocus activities. Healing is directly related to the inner being.

According to the sages, a human body is a boat that carries the practitioner to the spiritual world. The simple fact is that when you have some physical pain, how can you continue your meditation calmly? Or, if your boat (bodily form) is broken, how can you cross the ocean to find the Immortal Island? Good health is a natural benefit of all types of qigong practices, including meditation. All high-level masters of any type were and are physically healthy. If such a master has an illness for some reason, the illness is under his control. I have included such stories and described them in my book, *Qi, The Treasure and Power of Your Body*.

The sages from different times emphasized the importance of good health because our bodies are the transportation that carries our spirits to fulfill our destiny. The Lord Buddha emphasized this point repeatedly in his teachings, telling his students that after they finished a certain set of exercises, they would become healthy, their skin would glow and become fine-textured, and they would feel happy. He pointed out that "if someone only practices being void for a long time, it would cause deficiency and the practitioner should eat some tonic food and absorb energy from the universe."

## Soul

SELF-EFFORT PRACTICE AND THE INNER BEING

The inner being that can be revealed by self-effort qigong practice is called "soul" in all cultures. A soul can be exercised and cultivated to different levels in qigong practice according to the records of immortals of all types. In the next sections, we will explore how qigong theory defines soul and spirit. Whatever terms are used, the well-known Daoist master Chen reminded people, "Even Lao Zi had to say that 'Dao' is the word he used to define something that he was not sure how to name. So we better not sink deeply in the terms of this material that is full in the universe."

According to Daoism (such as described in *Chun Yang San Shu* by Immortal Lu), Buddhism (described in the *Leng Jia Classic*), and books written by the ancient well-known Confucian scholars (for example, Shao Kang-Jie), a soul begins to enter a baby's body only at the moment when the child is born. There are no differences between the "ages" of the souls between a newborn and an eighty-year-old.

In Daoist terms, the soul is inseparable from the primary qi. Qi is an essential part of Chinese culture, medicine, and diet. The primary qi is the origin of life. To an ordinary person, when his soul leaves the body at the moment of dying, they are losing the control of their own qi.

**Young Children and Their Souls.** Because of beliefs about the soul in Chinese culture, a young baby's spirit is always protected with caution. Chinese people believe a young baby can see things that adults cannot. Grandparents do not encourage young parents to take their babies to dark places or to funerals for a long time. I remember seeing an incident when a little child was scared by something unknown. The grandmother took the child's unwashed shirt or coat that still carried the child's energy, and went to the place where the child had been frightened. I followed her but was told to watch from a distance. She walked around and called the child's name, saying, "Come back, my child, come back home with me." This activity was "calling the soul back to come home" because the Chinese people believe that the child's soul was scared out of her body and needed to be guided back. Interestingly, in the cases that I observed when I was a child, the baby would stop crying during the night and become calm again. Occasionally if calling the soul did not work, the next day the parents would give the child some herbal formula for infants. Are these simply superstitions? Or maybe it was a coincidence that the child was healed? I do not have answers for you. I do believe, however, that a baby is quite different inside from the adorable way she looks.

I had similar experiences with my own children. My three-year-old daughter was playing with her building blocks alone in the living room. When I went to the table, I found that she finished constructing a "building" exactly following a complicated set of illustrated instructions. I became excited and called people loudly, "Come and look!" My brother-in-law kept shaking his head and did not believe that my young daughter could build this beautiful "building" completely by herself. He thought I was cheating and had given her some help. Could it be at that moment that my baby daughter's soul performed wonderfully? A young child's "wisdom" can be explored in a tranquil environment. We all have the same mature spirits within.

Another experience was with my son. A couple of hours after I gave birth to him in the hospital, I took him home with me. The third day after my son was born, his father came home. He held my son during the quiet midnight and imitated what my mother did, making the sound, "en, ennn" trying to make the baby empty his bowel. My son imitated his father's voice! His father was quite surprised and made the sound again, and changing his sound to a rising tone, "en-en." The baby imitated his father in exactly the same way! I quickly sat up and listened attentively. The third time, my son imitated again his father's "complicated" tone that he purposely did in a lower-rising-down tone, "enn-en!" The baby did it again! The excited father began shouting loudly, "Come and listen! This little fellow is able to imitate my voice!" The whole family woke up and came to the bed. But surrounded by five talking people, my son did not repeat any sounds that his father made, nor did he ever imitate any sound later. Because of the quietness of the night and the fact that my newborn son was right with me, had left the noisy hospital immediately, and arrived at our quiet home may have been the reason that my newborn son was able to perform in such a surprising way. His soul had not been disturbed—unlike my daughter who was born with difficulty and was taken away from me for three days due to an injury on her head.

The puzzle is why after being disturbed by the outside world does a newborn's abilities suddenly retreat. This may be one of the reasons why, when a Chinese mother gives birth, a quiet environment is always requested so that a soul can come calmly? How are the body and the spirit related? My experience with my children has convinced me to believe that inside a baby, there is an "old" soul.

**Yin Moral Belief and the Soul.** The word, *yin*, comes from Daoism. Yin moral, such as good deeds done but unknown, is also a belief considered important in the practice of Daoism and Confucianism, especially in high-level qigong practice. A simple truth is that when you feel decent and help others, you feel good about yourself, do you not? According to Traditional Chinese Medicine, when a person feels good about one's self, the mind's state is at ease. In this condition, his qi circulates well, which is a healing process. To a high-level qigong master, this ease means that he is in control of his soul, or the fate of own reincarnation. One of the most important Daoist classic, *Yin Fu Classic* (陰符經) whose author is unknown, says, "To be good at cultivating morality is Dao, which is the essence of yang." This theory will be explained more fully in the section about the spirit.

**The Seed of Buddha.** In Daoist terms, the seed of Buddha is called the primary qi, the longevity dan. From the Chinese character for Buddha, fo (佛), you can discern the Chinese definition of Buddha. The character, Buddha, is formed from two parts: on the left side is a person and an ancient word for "not" on the right side. The ancient "not" is formed, in an interesting way, by three lines that are joined. We may think of the three lines as the three main qi channels in qigong practice. In high-level qigong practice, when the three main channels merge and become one (or has integrated with the universal qi), the qi in the practitioner's body has been totally changed into yang energy, which is also the qi status of an immortal. This Chinese character also shows how an ordinary person can possibly become such a superior being whom we call Buddha. Another Buddhist practice, *chan* (or zen later used in Japanese) reveals the same theory as the above. Chan is a quiet individual qigong practice through a deep and thorough understanding of the progress and processes made when the practitioner's body changes during meditation. The achievement is gained by awareness, knowledge and wisdom. The character, *chan* (禪) is formed by two other words, "to show" and "alone," which indicate the way of chan practice. Regardless of the type, all Buddhist practices (for example, the

Buddhist Tibetan Mi Zong) adhere to the belief that Buddhas and celestials are human beings themselves.

Many other Chinese characters, idioms, and sayings can express this strong belief in man-made Buddhas and man-made celestials because the origin of this philosophy does not derive from superstitions. The Buddha himself encouraged his students to challenge his lectures so that his students could use their own wisdom to seek the truth. In the *Buddhist Classic*, the Buddha taught,

> *Monks, nuns, and scholars, you should think and question about what I said to you about the way you refine the gold, to cut, and to forge. You should not just follow blindly because you respect me.*

Although an intelligent Buddhist practitioner can practice alone and come to understand xing (nature) or longevity, the achievement of Daoist immortal status such as living for more than one hundred years is not guaranteed. Her continuing practice, however, ensures good health, even a long life. An improvement in the practitioner's health is a basic achievement of practicing Buddhism.

The book, *Travels of Marco Polo*, also includes descriptions of some qigong phenomena demonstrated by qigong masters in front of the Emperor, Kublai Khan of the Yuan Dynasty. Marco Polo witnessed those phenomena himself when he served as an official in the Forbidden City during that dynasty.

**The Invisible Teachers of Tibet.** An invisible spiritual teacher originally guided a Grand Master of Tibetan qigong, Wang Zi-Shen. Wang told me how he found his real live teacher during his first trip to Tibet. When he was staying in a small, crude hotel, he met a group of monks in a monastery next to his hotel. The head monk, the Master Monk offered him some food with his "dirty" hand. Wang ate the food because he knew that the master's hand was not only cleaner than an ordinary person's, but carried good qi that would only benefit him. Wang conversed with the Master Monk who told him in broken Chinese where he should go to find his teacher. The next day, Wang woke up and went to visit the monks again. He went the same place, but found no monastery—nothing was there. He asked a clerk but was told that there were no other buildings nearby—the hotel itself was in the middle of nowhere! Master Wang has been teaching qigong in Los Angeles in the United States since 1994. Once in a while, he takes his students to Tibet to visit and learn from the teachers who live in the mountains.

**Reincarnation and the Soul.** In Buddhist terms, soul is related to "reincarnation." Reincarnation is a theory that has become entwined with Daoism and Confucianism because they share the same fundamental theory of the origin of life. Rinpoche Luosangtudanpai explained in his book, *The Differences between Buddhism and Tibetan Buddhist Mi Zong*, that "there is a world full of lives that naked human eyes cannot see, just as they cannot see electrical and biological energy fields...Human lives, like all living things, live in continuous streams. The human bodies are formed by the body forms given by the parents; and *yi shi* (consciousness, awareness, knowledge) that form the spirit streams."

Reincarnation is defined in Chinese culture as a state in which all people are reborn based on their preordained fates due to what they did in their previous lives. Their fates can, however, change due to the deeds they perform in their present lives. All Chinese customs, including festivals, provide much information about how human beings are related to the spiritual world.

Let me use Chinese funeral arrangements as an example. Monks, nuns, or Daoists chant at a funeral to guide the dead person's soul to go to the right place, to avoid wandering away, and the like. When I was a child, I watched several such funerals. When I saw a pole hanging out at the gate of a house with white cutting paper on top of it, as a flag, I knew someone had died in that house. The flag, which was used to call back the dead person's soul, was named the "keeping the soul flag." It is also used to call back the soul that could wander away. In Daoist terms, this calling back helps avoid the dead person's primary qi from scattering or floating to someplace else. On each seventh day of the funeral period, a commemorative activity takes place, and the dead would usually be buried after forty-nine days. If the dead body had to be buried earlier than the forty-ninth day, the family still would follow the rule of seven and bury the dead on a seventh day. The last activity occurring before they buried the dead would fall on the night of the forty-ninth day. On this night, the son (or if there was no son, a young male of the same generation) would carry the white flag on his shoulder followed by the entire wailing family and relatives to burn the paper "money," paper-made "property, " even some paper-made "servants," and the flag. When burning the paper items, the son would tell the soul of the dead that her body could "go home and rest with the ancestors." This burning was done to prepare a comfortable life for the dead in the "yin world," a place where only souls go. According to Buddhist beliefs, in the yin world, all souls of the dead people had to wait for their trial or assignments. They were evaluated according to what they did when they were alive in the yang world, which is for living people.

In Chinese culture, heaven and hell are defined differently from the Western cultures. Heaven, in Chinese culture and also in qigong theory, refers to different levels or dimensions. Hell, as a Buddhist term, means only the lowest level in the yin world where very bad, hopeless people's souls who can never reborn as human beings reside. The rest of the yin world is reserved for common people's souls to be reborn as human beings. According to reincarnation, judges decide whether souls are "rewarded" and born into rich families or to poor families. Because of this belief, when some Chinese people quarrel, they often say, "Do some yin-good deeds for the sake of your next life and your children!" Yin also means invisible. The yin-good deeds include the good deeds that someone has done, yet they remain unknown; moral integrity also creates good karma.

The highly respected well-known qigong master and scholar, Nan Huai-Jin, says every human being is born with a Buddha nature. If a dying person holds his attention at the heart and thinks of Buddha, his soul knows where to go. Master Nan adds that he often sees souls walking by him, those who cannot control their spirits. They stare blindly and walk in a hurry. He saw a soul jump into a pigpen and be born a pig due to his previous life of crime; he saw a soul bump in a shabby house and be born a baby; another soul went into a big, nice house, and so on. Such souls are the people who do not have control of their inner being.

I have met different qigong masters who are believed to be able to communicate with souls. Here are some true stories about the soul. The masters whose stories are given here have asked that their names not be given. In the late nineties, I personally saw a three-month-old baby in the United States who continued crying ever since he was born, despite being examined by doctors from different hospitals who all said there was nothing wrong with the child. In contrast, two Chinese grand qigong masters could tell that this child had an inborn problem by simply looking at him; they added that there was no way to heal except by time. By "sending a soul" over from a different city 170 miles away, one of the qigong masters helped the baby sleep quietly for one night. The young parents had their first quiet night's sleep since their baby was born. But that was all the master could do. Another story happened several years ago after I told a grand master about the mice problem in our house. He sent his spirit from two thousand miles away to "talk" to the mice. Since that night, we no longer have mice running around in our house as my whole family can tell you. In the 1990s, a well-known Chinese writer, Keh Yun-Lu, wrote about his interviews with some Chinese children who developed their extrasensory abilities under the guidance of their qigong teachers. These children all said that while they usually "saw" one person standing behind an individual, they "saw" several people standing behind some grand qigong masters.

## Spirit–Shen

### DEFINING SHEN/SPIRIT IN CHINESE

Before you read the following section, it may be helpful if you know more about the Chinese word, *shen*, as it is commonly used in the Chinese language. For example, to mean the look in the eyes, one says "the shen in her eyes." To mean the feelings, it is, "the xin (heart-mind) shen." To mean the appearance, it is, "the facial shen." In a word, to mean either feelings or a health condition, shen is used in the description in qigong as well as in Daoist and Buddhist terms. Shen means spirit, celestial (immortal). Let me show you how shen is written. The word (神) is formed by "to show," and on the right side is another word, "field" (earth) but with the middle straight line penetrating the "field". The written word, shen, can be defined as meaning the spirit is no longer restricted to the earth—a person has become a celestial (immortal). In the Chinese language, both immortal and celestial use this word, *xian*. Celestial in Chinese is *shen xian*

(仙). The character, xian–immortal–is formed by a "person" and a "mountain," indicating a person who practices qigong in the mountains. In another words, shen is a refined human soul that has become very different from a regular soul. Shen is a person who has taken control of her own soul.

**Defining Po/Spirit in Chinese.** We use the Chinese definition of shen to mean the spirit. Other words can also show the different levels and sides of the human spirit. For example, when saying soul, the Chinese often say *hun po* (魂魄). In Daoism, *hun* means the active spirit and *po* is the calmness one associates with courage, a capability. These two words are also used to mean the English word soul. I have not found a suitable English word for po. Hun and po are inseparable because they also stand for yang and yin that is related to qi. "Daring and resolution" in Chinese is called the po strength. A person who has po strength is bold and resolute in getting things done. When describing someone who is capable of doing difficult feats such as managing a large company well or resolving a crucial situation, it is said he has the po strength. When describing someone who is scared to death, it is said his hun flies away and his po is scattered. The book, *The Definition of Dao De Jing*, written by a well-known Daoist Grand Master Zhen Yangzi, states that, "po is the shen of the xin (heart-mind)." The classic, *The Yellow Emperor Nei Jing* written 3,700 years ago, says that, "only when a body has both hun and po, is this body a living person. When qi is plentiful, the hun and po become strong; if the qi is weak, so will the hun and po be weak." Whether the hun and po stay in harmony with their owner depends on how the owner manages and controls his own qi. When this owner has drained most of his qi, the person becomes very weak physically. In this condition the hun and po are ready to leave, which is only the situation of an ordinary person. This is not the case of a high-level qigong master. A high-level qigong master has control of his hun and po, that is, his spirit.

**Yin Shen and Yang Shen.** The *yin shen* and *yang shen* levels are described more fully in the chapter about immortality. For the convenience of English readers, I use the yin spirit to stand for yin shen and yang spirit to stand for yang shen. These two levels of spirits can only be produced in high-level qigong practice. Both the yin spirit and yang spirit still have different levels that the masters can achieve in their practice and cultivation. Between the yin spirit and the yang spirit periods, there is a transition period, the *yuan shen* (primary spirit), being delivered. This process is similar to becoming pregnant and giving birth—much work, effort, care, and caution is required.

# CHAPTER 2

# Dao and the Practice of Qigong

In this chapter, I am going to introduce Dao. "There are differences between learning immortality and Dao," wrote a female qigong master by the name of Zhu Chang-Ya in 1938. She added, "To practice immortality, one begins from refining the dan; in learning Dao, there is no need to focus on the dan, but to work directly on merging the shen and qi, to return to origin from life, and to attain Dao. The approach all depends on the person's will." Hers is one approach to the Dao.

## Daoism and Qigong

The essential point of Daoism and its qigong practice is that all lives on earth depend on qi; qi starts lives. Through self-effort, human beings can stay healthy and prolong their lives by using qi, cleansing inner qi, and inducing internal qi energy. When a person's qi drains away, the soul leaves. Qigong practitioners, however, can protect their qi energy and can use it to reveal one's own spirits. This self-effort practice is called qigong.

There have been many sages in Chinese history and in other cultures that have devoted their entire lives to studying qigong phenomena. The sages wrote many books and transmitted their experiences to their students; the books and teachings serve as rich sources of information. I use some of these resources to you that human beings have powers that qigong can help explore, such as self-healing, prevention, prolonging life, revealing extrasensory (psychic) abilities, and more. The information in this book was chosen from the best and the most reliable resources I've found during many years qigong practice, over ten years of extensive research, and the lifelong reading of classic Chinese books about qigong and Chinese medicine. (See the reference section for a partial listing of the sources, most of which are available only in Chinese.) Yet I consider these resources far from being enough. I am not a "master," but rather a qigong practitioner, a little Chinese woman who has sincerely tried to bring correct information from China to the rest of the world. Please keep in mind that everyone has different experiences, even when "walking in the same shoes" because the shoes and feet are changing all the time. Sages like as Immortal Lu Dong-Bin who wrote 1,600 years ago have cautioned since ancient times,

> *Do not take a one-time appearance of phenomena as forever worshipping a statue...what is more important is to practice in order to prove the phenomena by one's self.*

The "practice" that he emphasized meant qigong practice.

## Qigong Practice and the Ways of Thought in the East

I have found that when high-level masters try to define Dao, they all say, "There is no proper word to define Dao, no fixed form or way for Dao...Dao belongs to all." Dao is not a religion, but a way of thought that is similar to philosophy and a practice that is much older than any major religion in the world. Dao is the foundation of the theory of Daoism and the Daoist way of life. I think that a qigong practitioner should not confuse qigong practice with any religion although they seem to share some common traits such as tolerance, forgiveness, kindness, love, and peace. A qigong practitioner should not confuse practice with the Chinese Daoist and Buddhist religions. Yet qigong practice comes under a religious name because both the Chinese Daoist and Buddhist religions have developed many qigong forms, a fact I have explained in my other books. In comparison with non-religious qigong practitioners, the Chinese religious monasteries have made many more detailed rules for monks and nuns, to obey. These rules suit certain personalities. If the practitioners in the monasteries follow the rules strictly, they can use the rules as "stairs," make progress, and eventually may attain Dao.

One underlying principle exists in all types of qigong practice: individual effort. The bottom line is, although qigong practice and

Chinese religious practices have some differences, their highest goals are all the same—to pursue Dao. The different styles of qigong forms that Chinese Daoists (monks and nuns) practice are also used by non-religious qigong practitioners. I am not a religious person, but I have always valued the essence of Buddhism and Daoism, just as I study and obey the valuable sayings of Confucianism. I prefer to learn and study broadly, and have the freedom to choose the best teachers.

## Sources of Daoism

Although Daoism is an abstract way of thought and, for most people, too profound to study, there have been great qigong practitioner-scholars who have re-defined it since ancient times in ways to make it easier for people to understand. Daoism is the word that is used by the earlier translators who translated the *I Ching* and *Dao De Jing*. In the following what I will bring you is my translation from other sources. The well-known Daoist expert in China, the chairman of the National Daoist Association, Chen Ying-Ning (1880–1996) was among the few who has finished reading the complete set of the *Dao Zang*—a complete collection of more than 5,000 books of Daoism. *Dao Zang* includes over 5,000 years of history of Daoism as well as the different practices from the later Daoist schools. Master Chen Ying-Ning possessed many writings that had been handed down and had many students. He defined Dao in his book written in the 1930s, *The Daoist Religions and Preserving Health and Longevity* as follows,

> These are differences between Daoism and the
> others...Unlike some other religions that encourage people to
> seek happiness after death, Daoism encourages people to
> value physical health and the body that can comfort and
> help the present life. Unlike some other religions that
> advocate the ideal great harmony of the world, but when
> there are advanced nations invading the weak nations, there
> will be trouble in the future. The fundamental theory of
> Daoism is to promote a nation to work on itself, and then
> the present world will be Heaven...Dao can be taught
> publicly; fa [methodology and rules] must be divided into
> three levels to suit the individual. The skill/methods will

*even need to be more specific in order for individuals to choose and to be taught Dao now differs between the different individuals. There is Dao for the natural law, Dao for political ruling and Dao for individual cultivation...Daoism is not limited as solitary self-practice and cultivation, but is all embracing...To study the five thousand years of history, we should know that Confucianism originated from scholars who came from Daoism. When you study them, you will know that in studying Confucianism the scholar can learn partially; but when studying and learning Daoism the person will accomplish all. Confucianism is good at maintaining the achievements of one's predecessors. Daoism is good at meeting contingence (changes). Dao is different and it all depends on the person's will. There is Dao that people follow to work in the society [such as the politicians who ensured people peace and good life]. There is Dao that people follow to work on accumulating jing and qi and cultivate [such as the immortals]. There is Dao that people follow to become doctors to save lives. There is Dao that people follow to bring a country to peace...To learn Dao in a political career one will establish peace; to learn Dao to command troops one will become a strategist. To learn Dao to govern one will be able to make laws to make the society better; to learn Dao one can become an expert on medicine and this is how Su Wen, Ling Shu Qian Jin and Zhou Hou were written [all are important medical books until today]. To learn Dao one can become an expert of the Five Elements, develop intuition, and so on.*

Chen has further described Lao Zi's universal outlook as well as his methodology in his book defining the *Dao De Jing*.

## I Ching and Qigong

Studying in order to understand how qigong works is quite necessary and useful. A smart student will find the core truth of qigong from many different books. While erudite knowledge can be used to deepen one's understanding of qigong theory, it can also become an obstacle to the path of pursuing Dao. One of the most important books and also a primary source to learn the truth of qigong is the *I Ching*. The book is perhaps too abstruse for most people to understand in its entirety. If you are pursuing your spiritual path, try to read the *I Ching* repeatedly and try to comprehend it. Even while there is no need to become an expert, the book can help you understand more fully how life, qi, and qigong are related. Reading the *I Ching* helps you understand the theory of soul/spirit because it is a book of "culture and social dynamics, a book of the kaleidoscope of life" as Grand Master Nan Huai-Jin wrote. When you read the translations from the different masters, learn from their different interpretations of the text. I believe qigong is the treasure of mankind. Modern science can help people understand qigong, and qigong can promote modern science and enrich Western medicine.

## Defining the Dao in the I Ching

Now let us see how "Dao" is defined in the 3,700 year-old book that is considered the fountainhead of qigong and Traditional Chinese Medicine (TCM), the *I Ching*. *I*, pronounced as "ee," means creation, a complete-whole, absolute with no relativity. It also means to change—to live, to produce and multiply. *Ching* (or *Jing*) means classic. In the *I Ching*, it says that "Yin and yang are Dao...Lives reproduce repeatedly and never die out, the same as the universe, the earth and as all lives." In other words, we human beings are born "perfectly abundant and complete" with nothing lacking. Because there is no one word to define Dao, the author of the *I Ching* used the trigram symbol, "—" to mean Dao. According to Daoism, the symbol of taiji (tai chi), the yin and yang originated from "—". Taiji means an infinite energy resource, the creature of ultimate and harmony that eventually returns to "—".

Before the *I Ching* was written in earlier ancient times "—" was used to define this profound theory in the Ba Gua (the eight trigrams formed by the "—". "—" has been an abstruse subject that the Chinese scholars and scientists have been researching and studying since ancient times. There have been many definitions for "—" by either scholar-masters or high-level scholar-masters.

In another Daoist book, *Notes on the I Ching*, it says "—" also means

*...tolerance and kindness. When the universe gains '—', it becomes clear and peaceful; when the earth gains '—', there will be peace and harmony; when gods and spirits gain '—', they gain power; when a person gains '—', the person will gain longevity; when one is hungry, if the person's mind focuses on '—', food will be supplied; when someone is thirsty, if her or his mind is at '—', water will be supplied...After one has mastered '—', other methods will no longer be needed for learning. The person who has gained '—' will be able to stand on the rainbow, on the Big Dipper...because we are all from the '—'.*

In Chen Ying-Ning's definition, it is stated that "—" not only means qigong practice and cultivation, but also means 'chaos,' the primary qi....The "—" is the pure yang qi [cosmic yang qi] that produced all lives, which is its 'De'–morality in *Dao De Jing*."

Let me end the discussion of the definition of Dao with a story from the book, *My Family's Teaching* written by Yuan Huang (or Liao-Fan). Yuan was a senior official in the Ming Dynasty. His position equaled the vice head of the Defense Department. He wrote about his own experiences for his children to show them why the fate of a person lies in his own hands. Yuan studied Traditional Chinese Medicine when he was young because his mother wanted him to be a doctor to help himself and people. But one day he met an old man, Kong in a Daoist monastery. Kong was of great age who looked young; Yuan thought he looked like an immortal. Kung asked Yuan, "You have the fate of being a high official, why do you want to be a doctor? I have the book, *Shaozi Huang Jing Shi* that is meant to be handed down to you." This book was written by the well-known Shaozi (Shao Kang-Jie), one of the best *I Ching* and Ba Gua experts in the Song Dynasty (960–1279 AD). Shao was considered an immortal. It is said that if one studies this book and masters it, the learner will be able to foretell the future in a very exact way.

Kong predicted Yuan's future for his upcoming imperial examinations: Yuan would make the fourteenth in the county examination, make the seventy-second in the provincial examination, and would make the ninth in the Imperial examination in the capital. Yuan took the examinations and the results turned out exactly the same as Kong predicted. Kong also predicted the other events in Yuan's life, including the official posts that he would get and the salaries. All came true but the last salary. At this point, Yuan began to have some doubts about the predictions. After another three years, the Emperor raised his salary that was exactly the amount that Kong predicted. From then on, Yuan became totally convinced about his fate. He no longer worked hard on anything because there was no need, he thought. He often practiced meditation.

One day he went to Qi Xia Monastery to visit a master monk by the name of Yun Gu. They practiced sitting meditation together for three days without lying down. Yun Gu was surprised at what Yuan had achieved, and asked, "An ordinary practitioner cannot sit for such a long time because he is often disturbed by anxieties and desires. But in your meditation, your mind state was at ease and peace. This is unusual. There must be some reason." Yuan responded, "Old man Kong has predicted my life and there is no need for me to long for more and work hard anyway." Hearing his story, Yun Gu laughed hard and said,

"When a practitioner cannot reach the clear state of mind of being carefree, she will be controlled by the qi of yin and yang. After being controlled, of course their fate is fixed—this is only the life of an ordinary person. But fate will lose control of either a very evil person or of a very good person. Hah Hah! Is that the reason that for twenty years you have been controlled by your fate? I thought you were at a high level! What Old Man Kong told you was correct. It was yourself who did not understand the depth. The Heaven only teaches people according to his nature, but does not force anything onto them. All depend on self-effort. A person's fate is in his own hands. You create your xiang. [xiang—read the falling tone—means the physical look that a fortune teller studies about this person.] There are no portals for either happiness or disaster, all caused by this individual himself or herself."

Yuan suddenly realized what he had thought was wrong. He changed his attitude. Yuan and his wife both worked hard to cultivate themselves and help people. He later was moved to a very high position and he was able to do more for people. As a result, he did not die at the age of fifty-three on August 14th as Kong had predicted, but enjoyed a healthy, long life. He was not sterile as Kong predicted, but had a son. When he died at the age of seventy-four, the Emperor Xi Zong wrote an inscription to be carved on his tombstone and honored him highly.

I hope this story has demonstrated that Dao shows us we can take our fate in our own hands. Our own spirits are always within ourselves and waiting for us to connect and explore. I have learned such facts in my own qigong practice. From my own experiences, I also think further that even if a person who has been abandoned by the parents or by the family (even if they can never find the birth parents), or being a foster child, or a lonely senior, there is still no need to be sad or feeling lonely. To be in a human body form has given each of us an advantage and a privilege.

CHAPTER 3

# Qigong and Modern Investigations

Before you read this chapter, I want to acknowledge that presenting facts and supporting evidence is the only way that medical practitioners educated in the practices of Western medicine can be convinced. I can understand that many Western doctors are still unconvinced by the fact that acupuncture needles stop pain because they believe that laboratory investigations still have not yet measured the qi and the qi channels on which the needles work. When a surgeon operates on a patient, qi is invisible to the surgeon. When a Western medicine doctor examines the parts in a dead body during an autopsy, the doctor will not find qi either because qi does not remain in dead bodies. Qi remains only inside a living person. Ordinarily only Traditional Chinese Medicine doctors can detect qi inside a patient. The concept of qi and qi channels still puzzles most Westerners.

Nowadays, acupuncture's status has improved somewhat, but qigong seems to have to wait longer than acupuncture to gain acceptance in the West. Even as I have translated the findings from laboratory investigations performed on qigong in China, the facts and experiments still may be looked at differently by Western medical scientists and Chinese medical researchers. These two different types of scientists and doctors are educated within two totally different philosophies. Western medicine originated from an industrial society that is based on technology. The concepts of qi and qi channels originated from Daoism, a way of thought. The essence of qigong, Traditional Chinese Medicine, and diet is to harmonize qi inside the body and with the qi in nature. The treatment modalities include herbal formulas, acupuncture, eating the right foods, using *moxa* to heat, *tui na* to free qi blockages (*tui na*, which superficially looks like massage, but is different in nature), and *gua sha* (using a piece of china or an ox horn to rub on the patient's skin as a way to release the toxic elements in the system). Ordinary Chinese people use all of these methods to prevent or take care of health problems. The methods help to normalize qi and qi channels. In the following section, I will describe how qi energy differs from the energies that the West has known.

## Qi Energy is Unlike Any Energy We Know

We have to understand that it is not realistic to compare and judge investigations on qigong in exactly the same way as a scientific experiment on a material. Qi energy changes in all people, including qigong masters. A scientific experiment in the laboratory can give the same results repeatedly. When a qigong master uses qi to do scientific experiments, the result can be different from an experiment done with instruments. The results of the scientific experiments done by one same qigong master or by the different qigong masters on the same material can vary because qigong varies from person to person. Qigong masters are human beings who have feelings and emotions that can influence their qi energy and its movements. The master's qi energy can be affected by health conditions, emotions, physical changes, overwork, or other factors that can influence the results of the experiment.

An example of variable results is applying qi energy to kill microbes. Different environments can bring about different results; some experiments may even fail. The results can change for every trial even when done by the same master. Disturbances such as flashing lights, noises, or anything that causes the master to be uneasy can even cause a powerful master to perform less effectively. In a disruptive situation, the master has to use extra energy to resist some negative energy from people nearby. The results also depend on the qigong masters' level of accomplishment. This is why the results of qigong experiments are usually so variable.

According to many ancient writings such as the *I Ching* as well contemporary qigong books written by grand masters, timing is also an important factor that affects qi energy. For example, when yang energy starts increasing at 23:00, the natural world begins changing due to the activity deep inside the earth that is caused by the sun during the daytime. The qi energy inside us follows such natural changes. For qigong practice, there is the best hour in a day; a best day in a month; and times during a year—such as on a festival day (especially the festivals according to the Yellow Calendar, the oldest, original Chinese calendar created by the Yellow Emperor)—when the positive energy is stronger. For example, on a full moon night, our qi and blood circulates more vigorously; it is a good time for qigong practice. On January 1st (in the Yellow Calendar), qigong practice is the least effective. Practicing qigong at different hours (and different places) can affect the results and, in turn, such factors may affect the qigong masters during laboratory investigations. Timing also plays a role in determining the best times to meditate (See chapter 8). Modern scientific investigations support the existence of biological clocks, that is, that our body does change at different hours.

Qi energy is different from other types of energies. Many qigong experiments conducted in modern Chinese laboratories show that qi possesses "thoughts", chooses directions, and controls degrees of power by itself. It also "knows" the right time to cooperate and when to retreat. Such evidence from modern laboratories is unprecedented. Qigong experiments repeatedly show not only what qi can do, but which are open to examination by modern medical science. For example, when a person is practicing qigong, the person's heart and brain's current would be at its optimal condition, something that helps all the organs work together in harmonious order. Why does this happen? When internal qi becomes active, the practitioner has saliva that is produced in larger quantities than previously. The saliva tastes sweeter and contains more elements than when they are not practicing. I have experienced this. When a qigong practitioner practices for a long time, they can feel plentiful qi inside, they become more energetic, and they do not need as much food as before. I have experienced this. No any other energy can function like this. Qigong is from the human brain; qigong activities are the practice forms designed by human beings according to their personal experience. That is why qigong has thinking ability, has the ability to control the self, and has adjusting ability. No any other energy has such ability.

Emotions affect movement of qi energy and its abilities. Some translations from sources such as *The Modern Qigongology* and the *Nei Jin* later in this book explain how emotions can affect a person's qi energy. Results from Chinese laboratories showed that when a person is enraged over a half-hour period, the level of blood cholesterol doubles. In contrast, when a person smiles and relaxes, the blood cholesterol level decreases.

The sources indicate that when a person was in a qigong state, she consumed less qi energy; as a result, the person became more energetic because of the increased quantity of her qi energy in the body. During persistent qigong practice, the qi will be continuously stored inside the practitioner; the storing of qi ensures the person stays healthy and rarely becomes ill. According to qigong theory, when the qi energy is kept induced and stored to a certain level, the person's potential will increase. Many qigong practitioners, ancient and modern, have had similar experiences. This is also one way qigong increases the effectiveness of the immune system. According to Traditional Chinese Medicine, when qi is normalized and increased, the immune system is strengthened.

This is why qigong is the ideal way to increase the immune system naturally, to keep people in good health, to remain beautiful and young; and to prevent diseases. Qigong is also the only way to help reveal a practitioner's potentials such as the ability to use qi to heal the self, and to treat others. No other energy can play this role but qi energy. Also because of the human within, qigong does not heal in the same way as Western medicine a concept that I explore in the next section.

## Qigong Healing Compared with Western Medicine

Qigong heals in different ways than Western medicine. In Beijing, the average life span of its citizens is 76 years just as in America, according to Professor Fang Ting-Yu from Beijing Traditional Chinese Medicine University. Chinese seniors do not take as many vitamins and undergo far fewer surgeries than American seniors. In the following section, I compare the different healing modalities from West and East to help you comprehend better the way of qigong healing.

Western medical treatment follows this route: the patients depend completely on the physicians to take care of their health. The physicians, in turn, depend on modern technology, drugs, surgeries, laboratory tests, and machines to find the causes of illnesses from external factors and fight illnesses off. More and more powerful drugs are created to replace the ineffective antibiotics or other drugs that suppress symptoms. The focus is on removing environmental factors that trigger problems by using chemicals, transplants, bypasses, or artificial organs and finding an element or certain genes that may help treat or prevent a certain disease. There is much more time invested and much more money continuously spent on such research and inventions.

Educated to seek help from machines, instruments, and drugs, Western medical practitioners find qigong and Chinese medicine incomprehensible. The results from their investigations, such as identifying the active ingredients that are found in an herbal formula or in a qigong treatment, still cannot explain exactly how an herb functions in an herbal formula and how qi works in a qigong practice. Several American researchers examining a Chinese ten-thousand-year-old lotus seed found that the seeds contain an potential anti-aging agent, thus illustrating that the Western way is to look for isolated elements in the seed. The Chinese way is to look at how the seed works on qi present in living human bodies. In fact, lotus seeds are called spleen fruit and have been used as an herb and as a tonic food for longevity in Chinese culture for thousands of years.

In Traditional Chinese Medicine, many herbs, such as gingko leaves and nuts, are used in cooking and herbal formulas for prolonging life besides treating diseases. But the herbs must be prescribed on the patient's qi condition and the ingredients must be mixed in the right combination. Qigong healing functions as the "right combination of herbs" and the "right diet" for many different individuals at the same time. Neither herbal formulas nor qigong healing can be tested exactly in the same way in the Western laboratory as when the scientists authenticate a drug. Why not? Take one example of treating diabetes. According to Grand Master Xu Ming-Tang,

> Constantly injecting insulin to "feed" pancreas only has made the organ "lazy" and weak and totally dependent on the injection. Temporarily the injection helps the patient, but it does not resolve the problem. As a result, the pancreas will become weaker and die sooner. But if patients practice qigong to make this organ function again and work by itself, then the diabetic can be said to be healed. In a word, the patient has to "wake up" his own pancreas first.

Master Xu's phrase "to wake up the organ" means doing this in the qigong way.

## TRADITIONAL CHINESE MEDICINE'S APPROACH

Traditional Chinese Medicine's method is to focus on each patient's qi. For example, to treat the same illness, an experienced doctor will not use the same herbal recipe for all of her patients, but will reduce or add one or two herbs on a case-by-case basis. Advice about diet is also patient-specific. For example, a patient but not another may be asked to eat the organs (but never the spleen) of animals to benefit a patient's organ. The thick skin inside the chicken's large intestine called "the gold inside the chicken" is effective in treating problems with digestion.

The seasons, geography, the individual's sex, ages and the causes of the illness all come under consideration by the Traditional Chinese Medicine doctor. A woman's headache is treated differently from a man's. A headache or fever is thought only to be a symptom, but not the illness itself. For this reason, the doctor will not prescribe painkillers, but soothe the disturbed organ that has caused the headache. When treating an acute swollen gum and tooth, treatment is used to soothe the liver first. To firm the teeth, the patient's kidneys are built up for the long term.

Traditional Chinese Medicine treats patients by working in two ways: first working on increasing the person's inner strength, that is, the qi (induces the immune system) and second by treating the diseases by regulating qi to adjust the whole system. Qigong can function in all the roles that the herbal formulas and diet function. Of course, qigong healing will be more effective when coordinated with herbal medicine and diet because all the three enhance qi. When the practitioner learns some simple diet and herbal medicine, the healing can occur more quickly. Above all, qigong healing is the main power.

## QI HEALING

Why does qigong play the main role in healing? This is because qigong practice increases qi. We call this increased qi the "qi doctor" within. The qi doctor gains the power to travel since "he" has become energized. He will go wherever there are qi blockages that have caused the illness. At the same time, the right herbal formulas and diet can assist the qi doctor in removing the blockages.

In contrast, a drug taken over a long time functions in quite the opposite way—the drug disturbs the qi movement and even builds up blockages. Although drugs are also used in Chinese hospitals in acute cases, as soon as the patient's urgent condition is under control, most Chinese doctors will stop using drugs or start using minimal doses. In my talks with several Chinese Western medicine doctors, I learned that they are all more concerned than most American doctors with the side effects from drugs. In 2000, the American media reported that there were fifteen million people hospitalized due to side effects from drugs—many more than people killed in car accidents. Another news item in 1997 reported that several doctors found that penicillin was failing to kill bacteria when they used it to treat their patients. Several American researchers reported that powerful drugs induce viruses to change into new forms that are even more virulent. Many doctors have warned against overusing drugs in the United States.

Unlike complications with drugs, qigong practice has no side effects, which only increases its positive influence. The best part of qigong healing is that qigong practice prolongs life in a healthy way. And qigong can be a life-long tool for taking care of one's own health. Qigong is more effective than drugs because it is used to prevent illnesses. Prevention is the fundamental theory of qigong, diet and Traditional Chinese Medicine. The philosophy of prevention by working on qi is a core common belief in Chinese culture because it originated from Daoism that is at least 5,000 years old. Beside all the above, qigong healing depends mainly on the patient's self-effort, which contrasts with the premises of Western medical care.

All ancient emperors in China between 4,000–7,000 years ago were qigong masters, diet experts, and herbal medicine physicians, as were all ancient Chinese physicians. Now, if a Traditional Chinese Medicine doctor does not practice qigong, he still uses qigong theory such as the Eight Extraordinary Channels or Five Elements Theory in their diagnostics and disease treatment.

Most of the Chinese scientists and medical doctors who were involved in qigong experiments are often qigong practitioners themselves. In the early 1960s, some Chinese researchers did numerous laboratory investigations on qigong with several masters. Unfortunately, the research results were completely destroyed during the Cultural Revolution. Since the late 1970s, other researchers and doctors like the president of the Navy General Hospital, Dr. Feng Li-Da who is also the president of the Central Immunity Research Center, together with her colleagues have done extensive experiments with qigong masters and patients. They have proven that qi is a measurable material, a kind of energy that contains some elements and special qualities that other types of energies do not have. Dr. Feng's book, *Qigong in Modern Science*, reports many qigong laboratory experiments and data. In the last chapter, I describe some of the qigong experiments in more detail.

Now you may be able understand why I say that qigong is a comprehensive technology and science that can be investigated by modern technology and science. Qi and qigong are an open door to the modern technologies and sciences. Most experiments on qi and qigong are still at a preliminary stage. In the following section, I give brief summaries of what can qi do.

## What Can Qi Do?

In the 1980s, Russians discovered that the qi given off by qigong masters contain eleven kinds of rays of electromagnetic waves. Grand Master Xu Ming-Tang has done several extraordinary experiments with Ukrainian and Russian scientists. Between 1986 and 1991, Chinese researchers discovered eight kinds of recognizable

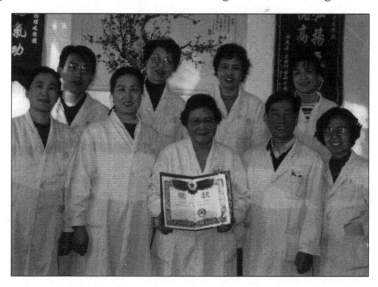

*Photo of Dr. Feng Li-Da (center), surrounded by her colleagues.*

rays and two unknown rays within the qi given off by twenty grand qigong masters. Even DNA can be changed. Dr. and Grand Master Yan Xin, who carried out many qi experiments organized by the government institutes and research centers before he came to the United States, was able to change the DNA and RNA's molecular structure, as well as the Roman spectroscopy of water molecules. Other unbelievable tests were done successfully from very long distances. Master Yan Xin's life story is told in chapter 6.

In 1986, at the Qing Hua University, professors Li Shen-Ping and Lu Zu-Yin used a Roman spectrum instrument (spex*1403 liza) to test the water, normal saline, and glucose saline processed by qigong masters. It was found that their Roman spectrum all changed.

In 1988, Qing Hua University, Hua Bei Medicine Company, the Chinese Microorganism Research Institute, and Chong Qing Chinese Medicine Institute all cooperated in performing qigong experiments. One experiment looked at how qigong affected microorganisms' genetic make up, or changed or killed the germs. Their experiment showed that qigong can change or damage the nature and quantity of nucleic acids. Qi of qigong masters contained material similar to ultraviolet, gamma, and beta rays.

Where modern science uses satellites to predict weather; a high-level qigong master can also predict weather and assist with the astronomical research as has been demonstrated in China. Laboratory studies depend on numbers and materials to get results. Qigong focuses on the relation between the mind and the body, between the psychological and physiological factors, the relation between the inner body and the outer world.

The invention of computers has allowed us to do many amazing things that we could never do in the past. Yet no matter how thoroughly and well-conceived a computer is designed, no computer can take the place of the human brain; no matter how advanced the technology is, instruments still cannot function in the way that qigong does. Only qigong can act in ways like the human brain does. No matter how advanced a computer is, it cannot improve human intelligence and memory by stimulating the pineal gland exactly the way that qigong does. Modern science has discovered that when a person is seven years old, the pineal gland starts a process of shrinking and calcification, and its function is one of the first in the body to weaken when a person ages. Qigong can slow the aging of the pineal gland and reverse our biological clock.

## What is Qi?

Here, I try to summarize the essence of qi by collecting the ideas from many qigong practitioners including my own practice.

- Qi is yin and yang.
- Qi is directional. It can go straight to the sick spot in the body.
- Qi has many similar characteristics to a human being: it has life. When a person dies, his or her qi is gone.
- Qi has thinking ability, self-control, and is able to adjust by itself according to an individual's need, or retreat.
- Qi is the organic conception of a whole.
- Qi can move around in circles or in both directions.
- Qi is not limited by distances.
- Qi is material, spontaneous.
- Qi can automatically organize itself and is self-choosing.
- Qi can store itself or preserve itself.
- Qi can pass inherited code.
- Qi helps people be more calm and intelligent.
- Qi can change the structure of cells, such as cancer cells, or the structure of nucleic acid in cells.

I hope I have given you a clear picture of the complete, systematic and comprehensive natural healing methods—qigong. My view is that the universe is still a large question mark for us, maybe forever a question mark for most people. We do not even know everything about our own planet. An American scientist once said, "We know more about Mars than about man's testicles." The Chinese ancient sages have handed us this human science—the qi theory that indeed we need to study and learn about.

> *"After you have crossed the river in my boat, do not carry my boat with you."*

> —*Buddha*

# CHAPTER 4

# Immortality

## Defining Immortality in Chinese

The practice of immortality is essential and crucial in high-level qigong practice originating from Daoism. The English word, "immortal" in Chinese is the "real human" (眞人), *zhen ren*, a term that comes from Daoism. I have not yet found the right English word for the qigong practice of immortality. The well-known Daoist physician, Hu Hai-Ya suggested that in order to be clear and avoid confusion, the ancient practice for achieving immortality should be separated conceptually from the early history of the Daoist religion (established officially in 141 AD by Zhang Dao-Ling who lived in 34–156 AD). Although some practices of immortality and Buddhism, as well as their philosophies, have merged and become entwined, there is also a principal difference between their ultimate goals.

Take the word, *xian* (immortal) as an example. Xian in Chinese culture and language means "never dies." This point of view is the opposite of the Buddhist view. Buddhism does not use the word xian, nor does Buddhism have a title like this. According to Buddhism, death is a new beginning of life, and no one can avoid death. But xian indicates that a person can avoid death. In the 1930s, the well-known Daoist master Yun Duanzi commented:

> *Immortality and going to heaven after death are two completely different things that cannot be mixed up. The immortal's rising to heaven means either the yang shen flying up to another dimension but leaving the physical body, or even leave-taking of her physical body. There have been records about these events, as there were a number of these immortals during each dynasty. In the practice of immortality, there is no focus on the next life, such as reincarnation in Buddhism. An immortal has moved*

*beyond the Buddhist 'six reincarnations' and gained the utmost freedom. However, it does not mean that one has to succeed in the once life time [what he meant is that an immortal can choose parents to be born.] But I am afraid that there will be some people acting in a way that defeats their purposes. Compared with the broadly promoted Buddhism, the practice of immortality is limited and requires a teacher. In the future, only immortality will be able to challenge modern science.*

## Practice of Immortality and the Human Body

As you have read in the passage above, the philosophy of immortality is focused on the present life, not only working to live much longer than a regular human being, but also avoiding physical death. Immortality is directly related to the physical body; good health is the foundation of immortality practice. The belief of immortalism is that human beings can live for hundreds of years, even over a thousand years and longer by practicing qigong and can become celestials who never die.

Briefly, immortality is to exercise the human body in order to return to youth, and then change the body's condition to go beyond earthly limitations—in another words, to preserve the primary qi that a person is born with. Primary qi forms the basis for a human being's existence and can be exercised and cultivated. By protecting and nourishing the primary qi, until the point of saving plentiful qi is reached, the body undergoes a profound quality change. All the channels in her or his body open up and join into one. The practitioner not only stays healthy, and can transcend worldly needs, such as food and air.

After achieving this immortal state, the next goal for the practitioner is to "fly" to the higher dimensions (or different realms in modern terms). This flying can either mean the physical body together with the spirit or just the spirit leaving the bodily form on earth. The type of flying depends on the practitioner's level, ability, or plan. To practice immortality requires profound knowledge, including Chinese medicine and diet. In Chen Ying-Ning's words, "Since ancient times, there are no immortals who cannot read and write." This is why Chinese medicine and diet originated from this longevity philosophy. The different branches of immortality practices all have leaders who were and are real people with access to the study of ancient books. Master Yun Duanzi mentions in his writing that there have been records about the immortals' ages, where they came from, who their teachers and disciples were, and who their families are. Immortality practices are not a part of any religion, not even Daoist religion; it is a "patent" of Chinese human science. You can read more details about this subject in my other books.

## Practice of Immortality as a Human Science

We can consider the practice of immortality as a form of human evolution with the immortal being the result of human body evolution. A poem written by Immortal Zhang San-Feng, the originator of Taiji practice, may help explain this theory succinctly and tells how a human being can become an immortal. (Zhang's story has been included in the end of this chapter.) "The Rootless Tree" was written by Immortal Zhang during the Ming Dynasty (1246–1403 AD). The poem, which I translated for the sequel to my book, *A Woman's Qigong Guide*, was carved on stones that are still preserved at the White Cloud Monastery in Beijing and at the Qing Yang Gong Monastery in Sichuan. Besides teaching the practice method, the poem says,

> *A human being's root is the head. It can be 'grafted' and grow in the 'soil' of the universe and become an immortal.*

Grafting here means practicing qigong and cultivating the qi with the help of an authentic high-level teacher.

The Daoist immortals also passed down techniques for refining mercury and lead into gold and silver to help them finish their journey to immortality. To use refined minerals and herbs is helps speed up the cleansing of the body. I have read about the phenomena in many ancient books. Chen Ying-Ning's disciple, the Daoist physician Hu Hai-Ya, said his teacher had succeeded in refining mercury to obtain silver before 1949.

## Shen Tong in Immortality Practice

The immortality theory may be too extraordinary for many people to believe. Reading these chapters will help you realize that we human beings can reveal mystical powers and become infinitely resourceful; this ability is called *shen tong*. Note that gaining great shen tong does not necessarily mean that the master has attained Dao. Also, gaining some shen tong does not ensure immortality. Any human being can explore shen tong. Animals, such as dogs who sniff for drugs, have low-level shen tong. A devil or false master can have explored some shen tong. A true master, who has achieved immortality, has attained Dao and has revealed a high level of shen tong although he may not show it. The difference between masters who have attained Dao and those who have run counter to Dao lies in whether they work on their xin (heart-mind) and are kindly to people. I have met and read stories of young Chinese masters who have revealed phenomenal power and whose teachers were high-level masters.

The immortals often help people in secret ways. A common Chinese saying is, "Those who show what they are capable of doing may not be the real immortals; those who show nothing may be the real ones."

Almost all true masters hide their identities or appear as ordinary people; some may decide to go public. To such masters, phenomenal shen tong are skills and "side products" that they gain naturally, but does not constitute what they seek. Shen tong to such masters exists only as tools to help people. "Shen tongs are like the gold powder coating the surface of the clay statues in temples. Only an enlightened xin (heart-mind) is like a piece of pure gold," commented the Sixth Reincarnation Rinpoche of the Tibetan Buddhist Duo Shi Monastery and Abbot Duoshi in Gansu province in his book, *Answers to 120 Questions about Tibetan Buddhism*.

## Guidance from Spirit Teachers

As in the West where people use Quija boards or séances to "talk" with the dead, the Chinese have also used similar methods to talk to their spirits since ancient times. A Daoist school headed by the masters, Yang Xi (330-387 AD) and Xu Mi (305-376 AD) started this practice. They used boards much like the Quija boards to invite celestials from other dimensions. A few Daoist books were written this way such as the *Chun-Yang San Shu* attributed to Immortal Lu Dong-Bin. In some local villages in today's China, children still play a game and ask questions from a spirit. A qigong master, Ou Wen-Wei told me that he used to play a similar game at night in a quiet flourmill with other children when he was a child. The answers to their questions were clearly written on the floury surface of a large container. When he grew up and became a soldier in the army, he was re-educated by the Chinese Communists to become an atheist. But those games that he played as a child had left him with some doubts about his re-education. During the 1970s, the Red Guards locked him in solitary confinement for eight months near a quiet area in the woods. That period started his twelve-year extraordinary experience with his spirit-teacher. Master Ou had had only a junior high school education and had never learned qigong before his invisible teacher came to him. His "teacher" controlled him when he refused to take his orders, and taught him human history, qigong theory, and some science. This spirit-teacher also changed Master Ou's body quality and helped his body explore potentials such as healing and extrasensory powers. Master Ou can sense the physical feeling of another person. When Master Ou stayed with us for about two weeks, I could tell that his body quality was changed completely—from an ordinary person's body into a body that usually takes many years of intelligent qigong practice to gain. The spirit-teacher never allowed Ou to "see" who he was and taught him through his voice. His spirit-teacher told him that human beings and all other living things on our planet were formed by the same elements, but only in different forms and structures. It should not be so strange after all that modern scientists who are unraveling the genetic code to defeat diseases have discovered that plants and animals share many genes with us human beings.

Master Ou's teacher also told him that human beings were the only ones whose inner beings were high-level spirits; only five kinds of animals (for example, the turtle, snake, or fox) have the potential to become lower level spirits. There are several fascinating classic Chinese novels about how these animals socialized with human beings and how they made effort to cultivate themselves in order to become human beings; they too could work on the higher level spiritually.

There are more qigong masters in China in recent years who have claimed that their extrasensory abilities or healing powers were not gained by practicing qigong, but rather were gained with the help of their spirit-teachers. An author, Mr. Keh Yun-Lu, observed and talked with a well-known young qigong doctor, Wu Jiang, who only needed to talk with patients during his treatments. People lined up and waited to see Dr. Wu. His work garnered much praise and thanks from patients for having cured their illnesses and improved their health. Dr. Wu told Mr. Keh how he treated his patients—there was a woman's voice talking in his head that guided him in diagnosing and treating the patients. This voice had a Beijing accent, which was not Dr. Wu's native dialect. Wu grew up in south China where the dialect is very different from the Mandarin dialect used in Beijing.

I once hosted a native African healer, Erice Yao Vermanns in our house and attended his workshop that he taught on using energy to heal others. From our conversations, I understood that Erice knew very little about Daoism, nor had he any formal education. He could not read and write, but his personal philosophy had much in common with Daoism. His methods of healing and his energy were also similar to those of several Chinese qigong masters that I have met. Erice also learned from an invisible female spirit who taught him by voice.

Qigong healers like Master Ou, Dr. Wu, and Erice Vermanns all learned qigong theory in reverse, that is, from the movements of qi inside their own bodies first, then from practice, and finally from books. Could the voices of the teachers of Master Ou, Dr. Wu, as well as Erice come from those who are called immortal—*zhen ren*, which means the "real human" as the Chinese language defines high-level qigong masters?

## Spirit Types

Before you read the information about the yin spirit (*yin shen*) and yang spirit (*yang shen*) that play an important role in refining souls, let me briefly introduce these terms. These terms are not Buddhist, but rather they are Daoist. Nevertheless, these terms refer to both the Buddhist and Daoist high-level practices for refining the soul. In all the high-level practice, producing the refined soul depends greatly on the practitioner's self-effort. To attain the refined soul is the same as the other types of high-level practices. But the approach to delivering refined souls differs. The practice of revealing different levels of spirits is to allow the practitioner to eventually live in good spirits forever. This is the essential theory of the immortality practice that originated from Daoism. This theory has been supported by the success of many real people's experiences in prolonging their lives. Such a strong belief that a person can live hundreds of years, even more than a thousand years, may be hard to believe. There are reliable records that show how some celestials accomplished this feat. No laboratory results have yet proven that this theory is correct. Even if she is already a believer, the scientist herself must become a qigong practitioner and achieve a certain high level before realizing the truth of the Daoist immortality practice. I personally know several Chinese scientists who have changed their views of life after they have practiced qigong for a long time and have attained Dao at the beginning level.

My Daoist friend, Gao Cheng-Zi told me once that "In fact, yin shen, yuan shen, and yang shen are different sides of shen. The celestials, immortals, and Buddhas in Western culture are called angels."

In the following sections, I will expand on these ideas. Yin shen, yuan shen, and yang shen are the three levels in a qigong master's journey that help him achieve immortal status.

YIN SHEN—INVISIBLE SPIRIT AND IMMORTALITY

The words, *yin shen* mean invisible spirit. Yin spirit is the refined, exercised soul that is a "product" of qigong practice. *Yin* means invisible, because a soul is also invisible which, in Chinese, is their shared meaning. A regular soul, however, is only partly related to the yin spirit level because it has no training or awareness. A soul fears the sun; a yin spirit cannot stay under the sun for a long time according to Daoist experts Chen Ying-Ning and Grand Master Xu Ming-Tang. According to many ancient books written by well-respected masters, most souls of dead people have no self-control, but a yin spirit of a qigong practitioner can be totally under self-control (except those who prematurely deliver their own souls hoping to advance their practices). Many qigong practitioners in China as well as in other countries can send their yin spirits to travel away from their physical bodies. Many can even travel to other planets or so-called cosmic dimensions however far the master's achieved capabilities can take them. Being able to send out the yin spirit does not necessarily mean a master who has achieved immortality; they must still practice qigong to advance to this stage. Masters can cultivate and exercise their yin spirit to reach higher and higher levels.

## Yuan Shen—Primary Shen and Immortality

The *yuan shen* is the product of the practitioner's self-effort and wisdom, just like a child. This spiritual baby can be produced in either a male or a female qigong master. His being is delivered because the practitioner has saved plenty qi and refined the jing into qi, and further refined the qi into this primary spirit. According to masters who have had such experiences, the yuan shen is said to look lovely. The yuan shen can be playful around the practitioner and is under control of his "parent." From this level, this master continues his practice to raise the yuan shen child with great care into an "adult," which is the yang spirit. The length of time this process takes depends upon the practitioner's wisdom and willpower.

A poem written by Immortal Zhang San-Feng may tell you about some of this process. I have translated his biography in the section about the eight immortals. The poem says,

> Something funny happened that made me laugh,
> That a man can become "pregnant" and deliver a baby!
> The "baby" was produced from my own essence and blood
>    integration,
> Who are the wonderful "husband and wife" inside me.

The baby mentioned in the poem represents the beginning period of the yang shen level, called the yuan shen (the primary shen).

With cultivation and practice, you may gain the power to reach the yang spirit level some day. When you reach this level, there are still more stages to achieve.

These masters then either progress on the path of becoming a celestial and a Buddha or they remain an earth immortal. Most sources support this theory although a few believe that yuan shen should come after the yang shen level.

## Yang Shen—Visible Spirit and Immortality

Although I have met numerous masters who have achieved the different levels of yin spirit, I do not have any personal experience to share with you about the yang spirit masters. Nor do I believe or am sure if I have met a master who has achieved the yang spirit level.

What I would like to do is not to discuss yang spirit masters, but to pass on what I have read in several authoritative books. Before you read the rest of this section, let me explain the words, *yang* and *tian xian*. Yang means "rising," "the sun,"and also refers to the positive energy of electricity. *Tian* means "the sky," "the heaven." The two words together, *yang shen*, mean visible spirit

Yang shen is a soul that has become purified into cosmic yang, that is, the soul has been completely merged with qi and jing. This is a high level achievement in qigong practice, though it comprises different levels depending on the progress that the master has made. According to a book written by Nan Huai-Jin, the half closed eyes of statues of Buddha found in temples indicate the yang shen level of practice. At this level, the master's spirit can be visible as a real physical self, whenever she wants to show you herself. Such a master can "separate" themselves into not just two, but to many beings. According to qigong theory, masters who have achieved the yang spirit level train themselves to increase their abilities to reach the highest levels—eventually, the pure-yang (the cosmic yang) state.

These masters have become those superior beings that we call celestials, or zhen ren (the real humans in Chinese). Some of them become higher level beings; people call them Buddhas. At this level, such a master can split one into two or more beings.

After attaining Dao, continuous practices help immortals move to different levels of dimensions. All of these achievements come from their own efforts in their qigong practice. The well-known Daoist master Yun Duanzi wrote in his book, *The Daoist Religion and Preserving Faith*, that

> To cultivate and exercise one's soul out requires much
> practice, like a woman carrying a baby, and also requires
> much work. If someone happened by luck to succeed
> exercising her own soul out by practicing only visualization,
> that soul would not have gone through the material exercise.
> Such a soul is not able to leave from the top of the head.
> Although in terms of immortality, it is also called "yin
> shen," it is completely useless.

The important ancient Chinese qigong books originating from Daoism that I have studied all emphasize the same philosophy as in

*Dao De Jing* by Lao Zi, "A person's fate in his own hands, but not heaven."

## Types of Immortals

### GHOST IMMORTALS—GUI XIAN

According to Daoist terminology, the practictioner who are at the lowest level of the immortals on earth are called "ghost immortals." The character in Chinese is *gui*—*ghost* (鬼) is formed by a field in the middle, a stroke in the top corner, and a human with a zigzag under the field. This character says when a gui reached beyond the field, she has become a *gui xian*. Their souls are different from regular souls because they can control their own actions, unlike a regular soul. The ghost immortals are souls who are able to cultivate and practice to a high degree on the earth. They remain invisible as the regular souls and differ totally from regular souls—they are their own masters and can do extraordinary deeds; they also help people. They can communicate with the other human immortals that are at higher levels. The ghost immortals can continue to practice and cultivate to achieve the status of a human immortal (that is, be reborn or borrow a body) or they can remain invisible to work on the next higher level, that of the heavenly immortals.

### HUMAN IMMORTALS—REN XIAN

Qigong practitioners who have gone beyond the level at which they have control of their yin spirits, they can continue practice to become different levels of immortals, such as the lower level of immortal called *ren xian* (人仙), the human immortals. Though the ren xian masters live on the earth, their yin spirit can travel anywhere they want. These masters do not become ill, nor do they age, and they can live many years longer than ordinary people. Their skins look young and their hair turns dark again. According to Hu Hai-Ya, the student of the well-known Daoist expert Chen Ying-Ning, if the masters' hairs still remain white although their skin becomes young and shiny, they are not real immortals yet. There are many qigong practitioners in China who have reached this level. The human immortals continue their qigong practice and cultivation. Their bodies become adaptable to any weather condition, hot or freezing cold, and they no longer need food and drink. They have become the higher level immortals—the earth immortals. But they still have to live on earth. This theory is the same in any type of qigong practice.

### HEAVENLY IMMORTALS—TIAN XIAN

Masters who have completed the yang shen practice are called heavenly immortals, *tian xian* (天仙). Not many of us can achieve this yang shen level. According to the well-known Daoist Chen Ying-Ning's lectures, there were quite a few such masters whom he personally knew, but none of them had demonstrated any magic powers for him. "Maybe," he added, "they were men of great wisdom who often appeared slow-witted."

## Achieving the Celestial and Buddha Levels

Not very many masters can achieve the celestial and Buddha levels. This is also why not many masters are called celestials. But many celestial masters are among us. "A celestial and a Buddha is only man-made," said Immortal Lu Dong-Bin in his writings. He is one of the well-known Eight Immortals that you will read about at the end of this chapter. To reach the yang spirit level, the practitioner attains Dao. The practitioner can, however, still achieve this feat differently. For example, if the practitioner has not completely gained the pure yang—if a bit of yin remains—his yang spirit is influenced by some emotions such as love or fear. This is why when practicing immortality, one needs to become free of cares and maintain one's morality. Because the path of achievements can differ, the final ways that the practitioner flies away can be of two types. One is that the yang spirit flies from the top of the head, leaving the physical body behind. The other way is to fly physically up to the other dimension. When the body of such a high-level Daoist master whose yang spirit has left is burned, there are usually no remains unlike the case of a high-level Buddhist master.

The lack of remains occurs because Buddhist practice takes a different approach from the Daoist approach. A Buddhist master can leave material remains in different colors, called *she li zi*, that resemble minerals. If there is a bit she li zi left after burning a Daoist master's body, this fact indicates that the Daoist master has practiced Buddhist approaches as well. See also my discussion about rainbow lights in chapter 6.

I end this part of my discussion with a quote from a high-level Daoist master, by the name of Ye (Ming Dynasty) who wrote,

> *I studied I Ching at an early age. I studied and studied, and when I got to the bottom of the matter, I began to understand what Dao was as well as my life. Jing and qi are material and changed by the soul that is in motion. When you repeatedly study and ponder them, you realize that a person can practice and cultivate physically, and even never dies.*

## Immortality Practice in Chinese and Tibetan Buddhism

Buddhism is not only a religion, it is also a way of thought similar to philosophy. The Buddhism that I describe is the Chinese style that has mingled with the Chinese ancient way of thought—Daoism. For example, the Tibetan Mi Zong also has roots in Chinese culture and was called Tang Mi (because it arose during the Tang Dynasty). The practice of Daoism was also shared by Tibetan Buddhism. If you look at the Tibetan flag that is used during important ceremonies, you can see the Ba Gua symbol on the flag. A Tibetan Buddhist school also uses a style of "pair cultivation" practice that was handed down by the great master, Tsongkhapka (about 1360 AD), an open minded and erudite scholar.

The practices and even achievements differ between Buddhist and Daoist immortality practices. Immortality practice is part of Daoism, and the Daoist religion includes immortality practice. Originating from the Ba Gua, the male Daoist practice is called *Qian Dao* and the female practice is called *Kun Dao*. *Qian kun* means "the world"; male and female are equally important as stated in the yin and yang theory. There are specific qigong practices designed only for females. There have been numerous female immortals who became well-known leaders of influential Daoist schools. They wrote many books. Daoist practice has domestic aspects and includes religious practice in the temples. They are entwined and integrated.

I do not know when and how that the Buddhist nuns officially were named second-class monks. Unlike female Daoists (also known as nuns), Buddhist nuns rarely became leaders of Buddhist schools. Even while there have been outstanding Buddhist nuns who attained

Dao at a high level, such as the only female disciple of Da Mo, Princess Ming-Lian and the later student, Princess Yong-Tai as well as a few Tibetan female Buddhas, Majilaya and Yixitsojie, they are not well-known. I did read in the earliest Buddhist classics and other books written by the Buddha's disciples that there were nuns among his followers.

The highest goal of Buddhism is to become a Buddha, and its starting practice directly aims at the xing (heart-mind, nature) and at the "void state (*xu* in Chinese)." This is unlike the immortality in Daoism that focuses directly on the physical body, in which the first step is to become healthy and gain longevity. Based on Daoist theory, practice for immortality does not just focus on accumulating qi inside the body in order to produce the internal dan, but using also the alchony, the outer dan made of herbs and minerals, a healthy life, and for preparing the body to be immortalized.

In contrast, the root of Buddhism is to work first on becoming unattached materially and emotionally in order to move beyond real life. The next step is to study and practice in order to become a Buddha. Unlike Daoist immortality, the Buddhist belief is that death cannot be avoided, but through reincarnation, one can become refined spiritually and eventually become a Buddha. The Buddhist theory that death cannot be avoided is diametrically opposed to the Daoist belief in immortality. The focus of Buddhism is not on physical health, but is based on understanding the reason why real life can be unpleasant, having compassion for other beings in the world, and working for a better life after death. To have faith" is a practice that is easy for most people and also has encouraged people to be kindly. When digging deeper into Buddhism, you will find that the way the character "Buddha" is written shows some similarities as the high-level immortality practice. My late father-in-law once sent me a saying from Confucius, "We come into this world crying while those around are smiling. We leave this world smiling while those around us are crying" which shows the mingling of the Buddhism and Chinese philosophies. A common Chinese saying is, "Everyone is born a Buddha." As defined in qigong theory, we all have Buddha nature, or the seed of a Buddha within.

In all types of qigong theory, when a human being has total control of her own energy, the qi, and one's own spirit, no matter whether the practitioner is a Daoist or Buddhist, her health and life is under one's own control and mystical power can be achieved.

Let me tell you a story about a Buddhist super power. A Chinese master monk, by the name of Hai Deng, not yet a Buddha, but well-known for both his qigong and martial arts, passed away in the late 1980s. It was said that he meditated without sleeping for over sixty years. During the Cultural Revolution, the Red Guards destroyed his large monasteries, but dared not go close to the small room where he was sitting. It was said that he could use witchcraft. When Master Hai Deng was in his eighties, he could still stand upside down on his index and middle fingers or on one thumb. He came to visit the United States years ago at the age of eighty seven. His students demonstrated some stunning martial arts in New York.

There are other similarities in such high-level practice for Daoist immortality and Buddhism. Often high-level masters hide their identities because they want to advance their practice with fewest disturbances and unnecessary troubles. Many of their powers are difficult for ordinary people to understand, they are not for mere entertainment or performance. High-level masters choose the right students secretly to teach and help people when necessary. Regardless of the high level achieved or the type of practice done, the serious cultivation of xin (the heart-mind) is the key to success. Though not many of us can become celestials or Buddhas, practicing qigong will, however, bring us closer to our own spirits; that alone brings good health and peace.

## The Eight Immortals

Stories about the Eight Immortals are popular in Chinese culture. They are Immortal Zhong Li-Quan, Lu Dong-Bin, Zhang Guo-Lao, Tsao Guo Jiu, Li Tie-Guai, Han Xiang-Zi, Lan Tsai-Heh and Heh Xian Gu (a female immortal). Each has his set of magic weapons and power gained after long qigong practice. Now that I have described immortality and other qigong phenomena, these stories illustrate how far human beings can go with qigong practices. The following is a brief summary of what I translated from the *Introduction to the Daoist Holistic Zhen School*, a compilation from the White Cloud Monastery. Monasteries for the Eight Immortals are found in many places in China.

## IMMORTAL ZHONG LI-QUAN

Chinese people like to call him Immortal "Zhong Li." He lived during the Han Dynasty and came from Xian Yang City in the Shaanxi Province. One legend says that one day before his pregnant mother gave birth, a giant came in her room and introduced himself as the ancient Deity Shen Huangshi who told her that he would be reborn into her family. Suddenly, a shining aura appeared like fire spreading in the room, and a baby boy was born—a large baby the size of a three-year-old. His extraordinary looks showed his unusual background. He had a round large head with a broad forehead, thick, big ears, long eyebrows, deep eyes, and a large high nose. His facial and lip color were rosy, his nipples far apart, and his arms long. He did not cry or want to drink milk for seven days, then suddenly he spoke, saying; "I had a tour in the Jade Emperor's Purple Palace and my name is written there." When he grew up, he became a high official; he was assigned to be a general commander to fight the enemies who invaded north China where he was defeated. He then disappeared to Mount Zhong Nan. In the mountains, he met several celestials and learned from them. He practiced and became an immortal. He met Deity Dong Hua and learned martial arts and the secrets of evolving into a celestial being. Later he met Celestial Hua Yang, who taught him more. He helped Lu Dong-Bin in his practice to become a celestial. Zhong is considered one of the Five Founders of the Northern Daoist School. In most paintings, he looks free and relaxed, and carries himself as an ordinary man.

## IMMORTAL ZHANG GUO-LAO

Zhang Guo-Lao's stories were recorded in ancient records. He was a Daoist in the Tang Dynasty and had super powers. He lived in Mount Zhong Tiao in Zhang Zhou county and was believed to have lived several hundred years. It is said that he often sat backward on a white donkey that was transformed from a paper cutting (an art form) and traveled between Shanxi and Shaanxi provinces to teach people to be kind. At night, he changed the donkey back into paper again. The Tang Emperors sent invitations for him to appear before them, but he refused to go. Later, the Empress Wu Ze-Tian persisted in inviting him. He had to go but "died" halfway there and secretly returned to the mountains. Many years later during the middle Tang

Dynasty, Emperor Xuan Zong finally got him to the Forbidden City and wanted him to marry Princess Yu Zhen. Zhang Guo-Lao thought about it, but said, "No" by singing a poem: "To marry a Princess is like to be in heaven, which he loves but can only put dread in me." He begged the Emperor to let him go back home. On the way back, he died at Pu Wu county in Mount Huan. His disciples said he had become a celestial and went to heaven. The Emperor ordered a monastery to be built in Pu Wu County in his memory.

## Immortal Tsao Guo-Jiu

Guo Jiu means the brother-in-law of an emperor. Tsao was said to be the brother of the Empress Tsao, wife of Ren Zong, the Emperor during the Song Dynasty. The painting of Tsao portrays him as being different from the rest of the celestials. He wears an official robe and carries two jade yin-yang planks. He had a very kind and merciful heart, and liked a simple life. He was deeply ashamed of his brother who ruthlessly robbed and murdered people. He left his family and went into the mountains to study Daoism and cultivate himself. One day Immortals Zhong and Lu went to test him.

They asked, "What are you studying and cultivating?"

Tsao responded, "Dao."

"Where is Dao?" they asked. Tsao pointed to the sky.

"Where is heaven?" Dao pointed to his heart.

The two Immortals smiled and knew that he had learned the truth of life. They gave him directions and Tsao became a celestial too.

## Immortal Li Tie-Guai

Tie Guai means an iron walking cane. The legends say his real name was Li Xuan. There are many stories about him. Originally, he was a handsome strong tall man. One day, he told his disciple that he was going to meet Lao Zi and would leave for seven days. If his shen (spirit) did not return to his bodily form on the seventh day, his disciple should burn the body. He sat in deep meditation and his soul went to the meeting. Unfortunately, on the sixth day, the disciple's mother was in critical condition and he had to leave the monastery to take care of her. The disciple had no other choice but to burn his teacher's body. Soon Li's soul came back, but he could not find his "house"—his body form. In the woods, he found a man who had just died of hunger. He went inside and suddenly found the body had only one leg. Just as he was preparing to get out of that body, he heard someone laughing and clapping hands. It was Lao Zi who stopped him from jumping out of the body, saying, "Dao does not care about the outward look, this look of yours is fine. As long as your gong is plentiful, you are still a real celestial." Lao Zi gave him a gold band to hold the messy hair and an iron walking cane. Li Tie-Guai often carries a bottle gourd on his back when he comes to visit our world. In the bottle gourd, there are herbal remedies that have magic powers which he used to cure and save people.

## IMMORTAL HAN XIANG-ZI

Han Xiang-Zi often appears as a good looking young scholar with a long bamboo flute in his hand. He was the nephew of the famous literary giant and senior official Han Yu. It is said that in his previous life, during the Han Dynasty, he was Ling Ling, the daughter of the primary minister An Fu, and was a beautiful and very intelligent girl. The Emperor wanted An Fu to agree to let Ling Ling marry his nephew, but An Fu refused. The Emperor became angry and dismissed him. An Fu was sent far away to do hard labor. Ling Ling was upset. She became so sad that she died and her soul went into a white crane. Immortals Zhong and Lu went to help her leave the body of the crane and be reborn again as a boy in Han Yu's family. The boy was named Xiang Zi. Since both his parents died when he was young, Han Yu raised him. When he grew up, he wanted to be a Daoist but was rejected by his uncle; nonetheless, he went to Mount Zhong Nan and practiced Daoism. Again, he was guided by Immortals Zhong and Lu and succeeded in cultivating himself into a celestial. Han Xiang-Zi later tried several times to help his uncle learn the purpose of Dao, but Han Yu refused. Ultimately, the Emperor demoted Han Yu because of disagreements with him. On his way to his new lower post, a heavy snow buried him. After Han Xiang-Zi rescued him, Han Yu finally began to realize that the real world was only a place to learn about Dao. He later became immortalized too.

## IMMORTAL LAN TSAI-HEH

The statue of Lan Tsai-Heh often carries a flower basket. It was said in fact that he was Deity Big Feet who was born on the earth. In theater plays, however, he was often dressed up like a girl. According to legend, he was a traveling Daoist who liked to wear shabby clothes and a wide wooden belt around his waist. On one foot he wore a shoe and left bare the other foot. In the summer, he wore a heavy coat, but in winter he bared his upper body and often slept in the snow. His body would melt the snow into steam. He often looked drunk, singing to tell people to be kindhearted while clapping two bronze music planks. He acted as if he were crazy, although in fact, he was not. A crowd often followed him. People gave him some coins which he stringed together and pulled along on the ground, often losing some of the coins. He either gave the money to the poor or bought wine. Some people who saw him when they were children would see him again as adults looking exactly the same. One day when he was drunk and singing in a restaurant, music came from the sky where cranes were soaring. He stood up and said, "time to go!" and left his shabby clothes on the floor. He rose up in the sky in a beautiful robe and was gone. One of his popular songs was:

> *Dancing Lan Tsai-Heh, how long can this world last?*
> *A beauty's face is like a spring flower, a year flies by like a*
> *    weaving shuttle moving.*
> *The ancient people die with muddled heads resulting in*
> *    many more who have come to this world today.*
> *Riding on my phoenix in the morning I watch the green*
> *    tides ebbing.*
> *In the dusk, I watch white waves covering the green trees*
> *    and fields.*
> *Long lasting lives and scenes are only up in the above,*
> *Where majestic palaces are built of splendid gold and silver.*

## IMMORTAL HEH XIAN-GU

Heh Xian-Gu is the only female celestial of the Eight Immortals. There are many legends about her. According to the records she was born on the seventh of March in a year during the Tang dynasty. It is said that when she was born, purple clouds rose in the room and there were six auras above her head. She was an extraordinarily bright child. When she was fifteen, a celestial came in a dream and taught her how to take mica powder (a mineral). When she did, she began running as fast as flying. She went to the mountains far away in the morning and returned at dusk, bringing back fruit for her parents. Later, she no longer ate food, but ate qi while on pi gu. It is said that Immortal Heh could predicted the future. The female Emperor Wu Ze-Tian invited her to the Forbidden City. She started out, but disappeared along the way. Another saying was that Immortal Lu guided her to become a celestial.

The poem about her on the columns outside the White Cloud Monastery says:

> In the universe, the purple qi shows the magic power of
> Dao.
> Deep in the white clouds is where the celestials live.

## Immortal Lu Dong-Bin

Immortal Lu is the most influential immortal of the eight and is known by old and young alike. It is said he was a member of the Tang Emperor's family. Li was his original surname. After Empress Wu Ze-Tian seized power, he had to hide along with his other family members to avoid being jailed or killed. He went to the mountains and changed his last name to Lu. Another legend says he was the grandson of Lu Wei, who was a high official in the Tang Dynasty. Before he attained Dao, he met Zhong Li-Quan, who lent him a pillow. Lu fell asleep on the pillow and dreamed that he came in first in the highest imperial examination and became a high official. He dreamed he married a beautiful wife and had a nice family for ten years. Then he offended the Emperor and was punished by being sent far away from his family, losing his family and money. At that moment, he woke up from his dream, and he saw the rice soup that Zhong was cooking before he fell asleep was not done yet. Suddenly, he realized how short and unfortunate a person's life on the earth could be. He begged Zhong to teach him how to live beyond mortal life. Zhong tested him with money, life and death, irritation, love, poverty, and hardships during ten kinds of testing. Nothing shook Lu's determination to pursue Dao. Zhong taught him the Jin Ye Da Dan and Ling Bao Bi Fa, and Lu gained phenomenal power. One day, Lu met the Deity Fire Dragon, who taught him more. Immortal Lu learned that practicing Daoism was also the only way to cultivate the highest level of Dao; one had to let go of greediness, anxieties, longings, and disturbed emotions. He applied himself to cultivating Dao and vowed to help and save people around the world. He finally attained a very high-level Dao. It is said that he often traveled and changed into different persons to help people. He even helped several others become celestials. There are many moving and interesting stories about him. People called him Immortal of the Sword, Immortal of Poetry, and Drunken Immortal because he was a very good martial arts master, a great poet and literati, and loved to drink wine. He was considered to be one of the five founders of the Northern Daoist School. Many of Immortal Lu's writings have been passed down, including the whole set of forms for female qigong practitioners. On his birthday, the 14th of April, a large ceremony is held in his monastery.

The poem about him on the pole outside the White Cloud Monastery says:

> One dream on the pillow laid bare the truth of one thou
> sand years of lives that are only empty dreams.
> Practiced Nine-Turning Dan and succeeded in becoming a
> celestial, he survived ten thousand calamities.

## IMMORTAL QIU—FOUNDER OF THE DRAGON GATE

Because Immortal Qiu became the Abbot of the White Cloud Monastery in the Yuan Dynasty and passed away there, the White Cloud Monastery has been considered by the Daoists to be the original place of the Dragon Gate Daoist School. Immortal Qiu, whose given name was Chu-Ji, was born in 1148 and died in 1227 at the age of eighty. (Chinese count the year before the person is born as the first year of life.) The records say when he passed away, the fragrance in the monastery area lasted for days. He was from a well-known family in Qi Xia county in the Deng Zhou area of the Shandong province. As a child, he was known for his extraordinary memory and quickness. At the age of 19, he became a Daoist in Mount Kun Yu (southeast of Maoping City). In his second year, he went to Immortal Wang Chong-Yang's Holistic Zhen Daoist School and became his student. During the three years of study, Immortal Wang taught Qiu mainly one thing—to be humble. Before Immortal Wang left his bodily form, he told Ma Dan-Yang, the Big Brother of his seven disciples to teach Qiu. He had predicted that Qiu would become the successor to the Holistic Zhen Daoist School. After studying and learning from Wang, Qiu practiced alone in the Fan Xi

Cave in the Shaanxi province for six years and cultivated Dao with great concentration. He was known locally as the "Sir Palm-Bark Rain Cape" (the ancient raincoat) because he took a rain coat and a bamboo hat with him wherever he went. He went to the Dragon Mountains (southeast of Bao Ji City), practiced there intensively for another seven years, and established the Dragon Gate Daoist School.

In 1188, the Emperor of Jin Dynasty consulted Qiu on Daoism and asked him to perform a ceremony for blessing the Emperor's ancestors. In 1207, the Empress gave Qiu the important ancient Daoist records, Da Jin Daoist Collections, as a gift. In 1219, when he was living in Monastery Hao Tian in Lai Zhou, Shandong province, the Emperor of the Jin, the Emperor of the Southern Song, and Genghis Khan the Mongolian Emperor, all sent invitations to him, but he accepted only the Mongolian invitation. Taking eighteen of his disciples with him, they walked for two years to the west to meet Genghis Khan. One of his disciples, Li Zhi-Chang vividly recorded their trip and the meeting with the Mongolian Emperor. His book, *Immortal Qiu's Trip to the West*, is a rich and valuable resource for research in geography, astronomy, biology, and local customs. In this meeting, the Emperor Genghis Khan consulted Immortal Qiu about how to rule a country. Immortal Qiu responded that, "The fundamental rule is to respect Heaven and love people's lives. If you want to rule the world well and be successful, do not kill extravagantly." When he consulted Qiu about longevity, Qiu responded, "To ease the mind and not have excessive desires are the most important things." Genghis Khan respected Immortal Qiu very much and took his advice.

In the year of 1224, Immortal Qiu returned to Beijing where Genghis Khan honored him by naming him the Leader of National Daoist Religion. In 1227, Genghis Khan ordered a change in the monastery's name, from Monastery Tai Chi to Monastery Chang Chun in honor of Immortal Qiu's name who was also called Immortal Chang Chun—Forever Spring. Qiu taught that Daoism, Buddhism, and Confucianism are equally important and are entwined with one another. For people who cultivated and pursued immortality and attained Dao, he considered it important to work on the heart without desires. He wrote books such as *The Discourse and Information of Preserving Health and Longevity*, *The Guidance of Cultivation Through Da Dan*, and *The Collections of Ming Dao and Fan Xi Collections*.

Immortal Qiu's birthday is on January 19, and there is a celebration ceremony in the monastery on that day. It is said that on this day he appears as an ordinary person, such as a scholar or a Daoist, and that the lucky ones will meet him.

In the middle of the Temple of Qiu in the White Cloud Monastery, there is a huge container carved from an old tree's root. The edge of the container is covered with gold and on the side, there are eighteen words written by Emperor Qian Long. The Emperor permitted the Monastery to use this container to send to the Forbidden City for money when in need and it would be filled full. Immortal Qiu's body was buried under the container at his death in 1227.

On the walls of the monastery is *Dao De Jing* in the ancient plum-style calligraphy written by the well-known calligrapher, Gao Wen-Ju, during the Yuan Dynasty. The writing is vigorous and magnificent. When you look at it from a distance, the characters look like plum flowers.

Having attained Dao, he knows the secret of life and has won the trust of the Emperors

In order to stop the massacre he traveled far to the west to advise the Emperor

Another poem for Immortal Qiu that was written by Emperor Qian Long (the original writing is preserved in the White Cloud Monastery) says:

> *Live for thousands of years, no need of searching for a secret recipe.*
> *One advice stopped massive killings, showing that Qiu is a savior.*

## Immortal Zhang San-Feng—The Originator of Taiji Practice

In presenting the story of Immortal Zhang's life here, I used my translation from Master Zhu Hui's book, *The Longevity Gong*.

**Immortal Zhang's Origins.** Reading the biography of Immortal Zhang and his theory can benefit qigong practitioners in their practice and study. The originator of Taiji and Wu Ji Gong was Master Daoist Zhang San-Feng. He was the founder of the Wu Dang Daoist School, and was well known as a great qigong and martial arts master during the end of the Yuan Dynasty and during the Ming Dynasty. A Ming Dynasty government document records his life fully. Immortal Zhang San-Feng's original name was Zhang Tong. His family lived in the Mount Dragon-Tiger area in Jiang Xi province. During the end of the Song Dynasty, his grandfather Zhang Yu-Xian moved the whole clan to Yi Zhou City (the area near Shen Yang City) in the Liao Ning province. At midnight of April 9th, 1247, Zhang was born. He was the fifth son. He was an extraordinary looking baby with large, round eyes and big ears. When he grew up, he was tall and strong; his back was like a turtle's and his shoulders were like a crane's. He wore straight, long whiskers like ji (an ancient weapon about ten feet long with a long and sharp end.) He either ate a lot of food at one meal or went for months without eating at all. No matter how cold or how hot the weather was, he wore a raincoat or a robe all year round. Because he never cared about his appearance, he acquired the nickname of "Sloppy Zhang."

**Immortal Zhang's Early Childhood.** When Zhang was five years old, he had eye problems and his vision became worse day after day. The Zhu Chi (in some ways like an abbot) of the Daoist Bi Luo Monastery named Zhang Yun-An met him and his parents and said, "This boy has celestial being's nature and his bone structure is supernatural. He is not an ordinary person. But he has met some evil elements that caused his problems with his vision. To heal his vision, he has to be my student first. After I heal him, I will give him back to you." Since then the five-year-old Zhang stayed in the monastery and studied classics of Daoism, Buddhism and Confucianism. His teacher taught him the Holistic Zhen Daoist School type of qigong and martial arts. After seven years of study and learning, his knowledge and experience were widened rapidly. Because he missed his mother, his teacher let him go home.

**Immortal Zhang's Search for the Dao.** In 1260, when he was 14 years old, Zhang passed the imperial examination at the county level and earned the Scholar's Position (Xiu Tsai). He did not take further examinations because he was not interested in being an official. In 1264, when he was visiting a friend in the capital, the friend reported his intelligence to the Emperor. As a result, the Emperor gave him an official position. After Zhang handled his official business, he always went to visit Mount Ge Hong, which had been established in the memory of an historically important Daoist, Ge Hong. In the following year, first his mother died and then his father. Zhang took this opportunity to give up his position and stayed home to take care of his parents' tombs for a few years. (According to the law, the emperor had to give an official the time to guard his parent's' tomb when they died.) One day, a Daoist came to visit Zhang; they talked and discussed profound Daoism. The conversation kindled Zhang's enthusiasm and he left home to seek the truth of Dao. Since that visit, he traveled all over the country and visited and stayed in many well-known places and monasteries where the ancient sages practiced and cultivated Dao. He studied and learned in this way for thirty years.

Later he found the mountain called The Three Peaks with springs and trees in Shannxi province where the scene was pleasant and qi was pure. He settled down there. He named himself "San Feng Ju Shi—"The Three Peak Ju Shi"—a "Lay Buddhist or Daoist who practices at home." In 1214, Zhang went to Mount Zhong Nan (south of Xi An City) where Immortal Lu Dong-Bin practiced during the Tang Dynasty. He met an immortal, The Dragon of Fire, a Daoist by the name of Jia De-Sheng there. Immortal Jia taught him Dao. Zhang named himself Daoist Xuanzi and cultivated and practiced in Mount Zhong Nan for four years. Then Immortal Dragon of Fire taught him the secret of how to use *dan sha* (cinnabar) to advance his practice. In 1342 when he was 77 years old, Zhang went to Mount Wu Dang, studied and cultivated and practiced for another nine years after which he attained high levels of Dao. He was 85 then. After that, he traveled quietly in Hunan, Sichuan area for over ten years.

In 1359, at the age of 95, the records show that he went to the Capital. In 1359, in, he met Shen Wan-Shan in Nan King City and learned more about cultivating dan. After learning from Shen, Zhang returned to the Three Peaks and advanced his practice. He became famous for attaining Dao. The emperors at different times of the Ming Dynasty all wanted him to come to the Forbidden City. The first Emperor of the Ming Dynasty, Zhu Yuan-Zhang, sent out invitations several times for him, but could not persuade him to come. Emperor Cheng Zu sent senior officials Hu Ying-Xie and Zhu Xiang with the Emperor's retinue and gifts, and they unsuccessfully tried to find him for a few years. Afterwards, the Emperor sent Marquis Zhang Xin and the Minister of the Department of

Construction to take more than thirty thousands workers to build a Monastery for Immortal Zhang in Mount Wu Dang. It cost millions of silver coins. After it was finished, Immortal Zhang simply disappeared. In 1459, Emperor Ying Zong again sent officials to offer Immortal Zhang a high position, but Zhang did not appear. After that, no one ever knew where he went.

**Immortal Zhang's Beliefs.** Immortal Zhang carried out the Holistic Zhen Daoist belief that Daoism, Buddhism and Confucianism belong to One. He said,

> *A Confucian is gentle and compromises, practices Dao and helps the real world according to the right timing. To have attained Dao and know the truth of the real world is a Buddha. To hide the status of having attained Dao and help people is an immortal. They each have their own character and advantages, there is no need to debate about them. I have studied one hundred different schools and researched the three of them and this is how I have learned that these three belong to One."*

**Immortal Zhang's Qigong Practice.** Immortal Zhang studied the extremely subtle and profound taiji intensively, and observed the changes in the world and in the universe. On this foundation, he established the Wu Dang style. Later the style developed into the official Thirteen Movements that has been handed down.

To succeed in practice, Immortal Zhang San-Feng emphasized that one must "Remove the drawbacks [incorrect practice] of inflexibility [rigidity]." In his book, *Xuan Ji Direct Definition*, it says to, "Clear the emotions and attachments, get rid of disturbing thoughts." Only by doing so can the qigong practitioner cultivate and exercise his shen to return to *xu*—the void—and reverse the after-birth condition back to pre birth—the origin. He also said,

> *To practice qigong, one cannot hang on to the methods or experiencing, nor can one hang on to the non-methods or non-experiencing. The methods and the non-methods, the experiencing or non-experiencing that a person learns all come from the world after the person is born. Many Daoist practices cannot avoid introducing such common rigidities*

*or mistakes. This is why there are few who can holistically attain Dao. One should not hang on the 'emptiness' either because he will become the 'wan empty'—the 'hard-rock like emptiness,' which is a common mistake in many Buddhist practices. This is why there are not many who have cultivated and practiced into Buddhas. Dao cannot be carried out if the theory is not clear.*

# CHAPTER 5

# Qi and Life

## How Qi and the Physical Body are Related

Once, I met someone who told me that she had given up practicing the moving qigong form because she no longer cared about her physical body, but only practiced a Tibetan Buddhist meditation for spiritual purposes. Hers is a misunderstanding about any type of meditation, no matter what it is: the Buddhist Big Cart, Small Cart, the Tibetan Mi Zong, and Daoist, as well Confucian types. An influential Daoist, Immortal Lu Dong-Bin pointed out that "The most common mistake made in practicing to pursue Dao is to practice only for spiritual pursuit but neglecting physical health." The Lord Buddha himself also criticized some nuns and monks who committed suicide because they wanted to move on directly to the spirit level of practice.

### NUMBERS AND ASTRONOMY IN QI CULTURE

Qi culture in China predates Daoism, Buddhism, and Confucianism by a few thousand years. However, the number seven is special and related to spirit many different cultures. Numbers such as five, nine, and seven were always a part of the spiritual phenomena in Chinese culture. These numbers are all related to nature, and are used in the Chinese lunar calendar and the life cycle change.

According to Daoism, the Big Dipper, called the Northern Dou (*dou* is a large measurement utensil in Chinese), produces the *zhong qi*, the essential qi that produces a human life. To describe how a life starts, it is said that when the sperm and egg join, they receive zhong qi from the Big Dipper. The new life starts in the mother's womb, but is not yet a soul. This fetus in the mother's womb changes every seven days. After the first seven-day period, the new life's governing qi channel (which starts from the tail bone area up along the spine passing the head to the chin) will grow. In modern terms, this line runs from the diencephalon to the perineum (Hai Di acupoint). In my own practice, I have felt the movement through the governing (Du) channel and have also felt all of the other main channels flow basically in the way they are drawn in an acupuncture chart. Nevertheless, these qi channels are undetectable by modern medical science.

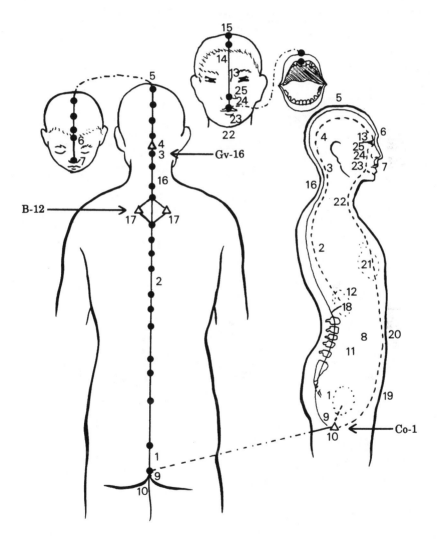

*The Governing Vessel (Du Mai).*

Continuing this seven-day cycle, after the second seventh day, the fetus grows the two eyes. At the end of the thirtieth seven-day period (according to Buddhism as well), the baby is born. Only at this moment, does a soul enter the baby's body from the top of the head. After the child is born, the child's physical changes still follow a seven-day cycle. A common Chinese saying is, "It is easier to save a seven-month premature baby's life than to save the life of an eight-month premature baby." No one has supplied me with actual scientific proof about this belief. I heard several real stories from people I knew when I was in China. Even the Communist government in mainland China has always given a mother 56 days off (seven times eight) after giving birth. After the 56 days pass, the mother is considered strong enough to work and the baby is ready to meet people.

## DEPENDENCE OF LIVES ON QI

According to the theory of qi—called vitality in Western terms—the lives of all living things depend on qi. When qi forms qi channels, we human beings become alive. This belief that a person's health and life depend on qi is strong in China because this qi philosophy has been rooted and intertwined with daily life. Many common sayings show how qi and the body are related in people's thoughts. For example, when mentioning a person is unstable and impulsive, it is said "his xin (heart-mind) floats and his qi is impetuous." To mention a dead person, the saying is "He has run out of qi, (or no qi is left)." When a person returns to consciousness after fainting, people say, "He has qi now!"

In Traditional Chinese Medicine, when qi channels are entangled up and form blockages in the body, the person becomes ill, or even mentally unstable. People can heal and gain good health by practicing qigong in order to gradually remove the blockages in their qi channels.

## QIGONG PRACTICE AS CULTIVATION

Qigong practice is a process of becoming physically healthy. Practice is not just doing the movements, but also involves working on the heart-mind at the same time—a process of cleansing her qi. In my A Woman's Qigong Guide, I have a full chapter introducing "cultivation" and there is little need to repeat the details in this book. Briefly, the cultivation process entails building up qi inside so that the practitioner gains the power to prevent illnesses and becomes mentally strong enough to peel off the layers that have formed on the heart-mind by the real world, such as by anxieties, emotional disturbances, greediness, and excessive desires. During this cultivation, the practitioner becomes closer to her inner being—the "real human," using the term from Daoism.

QI FIELDS

According to qigong theory, in the physical place where the high-level qigong masters practice for years, a strong qi field forms and gives off strong qi energy. That is the reason why in ancient times, the high-level masters all sought places and buildings where the immortals practiced. Several articles in Chinese qigong magazines such as *World Qigong* and *Qigong & Science* that I read some years ago stated that several modern researchers in China tested such places with instruments and found evidence that the qi-energy was much stronger than in other places. When a practitioner practices in a high qi-energy place and attains a very relaxed state of mind, her body can connect with the qi energy in the field. The articles go on to describe people who gained the power of intuition in such places. For example, an elementary music teacher, Liu from northeast China, gained her power when her qi energy happened to open up the "code" of the qi energy field and her qi energy "plugged into the switch" of that qi field. As a result, her qi channels were "tuned up" (processed for a whole month) and her potential was revealed at a higher level. For more detail, see the section below about intuition. I have included several other people's stories like Liu's in the chapter about qigong phenomena.

In the next part, you will read how our body is related to our soul and spirit according to qigong theory.

## How Our Physical Body and Soul/Spirit are Related

About how our soul/spirit is related to qi, Immortal Lu Dong-Bin told his student, by the name of Tu Zi,

> *The profound and comprehensive theory [of Dao] is in the hua [Read the falling tone, a magic word that means unlimited power of changing; sublimity, embodiment.].*

> *Without having an origin, one can hua to get it; without*
> *obtaining primary qi, one can hua to get it; without having*
> *the earth and the sky, one can hua to get them. With no*
> *human beings, one can hua to get them as well as to get*
> *everything. But this ability to "hua" cannot gain from xin's*
> *thinking, nor from feelings and thoughts. Words cannot*
> *describe this "hua" nor can inferences. It is the wonder of*
> *nature, but it is only a regular thing. To cultivate to become*
> *a Buddha, a person can be a Buddha; to cultivate to be an*
> *immortal, he can succeed because they are man-made [that*
> *is, by this individual's effort], which also can be effected by*
> *efforts made in previous lives.*

The word, *hua* (化) is related to the *xin*, the heart-mind. Let's us trace this xin and hua first through the ways the Chinese characters are written. The English heart and mind in the Chinese language are one word, pronounced xin, which is written in Chinese in a different way from the other organs. All the organs, hollow and hard, have a meat-moon as half of the characters, but not xin. (Meat here refers to flesh.) When writing the organ heart in Chinese, two words, heart organ—*xin zang*—an organ that will eventually die with the rest of the organs is used. The written "xin" hints that "xin" is not a piece of flesh and its writing tells us something about its nature (心). Xin is formed by one line curled with three little fire-like dots on the top. The three dots are defined as flames of anxiety. According to qigong theory and Traditional Chinese Medicine, xin is the fire element. Some people think that the dots also represent the three main qi channels inside a person. When the words are related to the heart-mind—such as emotions, feelings, and consciousness—all these characters have xin as half of their characters. Examples of such words are love, hate, irritated, upset, and understand. Even the written characters for these words can alert people about the conse-quences of being emotional. The word, to tolerate, has the word xin under the word blaze (忍), that is, to tolerate is as if having a knife above the heart. The word, angry, is formed by the word, to separate, together with xin; the combination means that the xin of an angry person is diverted.

Xin as it relates to the inner being plays an integral role in Traditional Chinese Medicine theory. When a Traditional Chinese

Medicine doctor mentions xin, he means not simply the organ, but the nervous system, the qi channels that relate to the heart as well as the patient's emotions.

Several Chinese characters define the relationship between the spiritual world and ourselves such as the character for brain, *nao.* (腦). Nao is formed by a "meat" on the left, its right side are three lines facing upward above a word, chimney. The three lines are symbolic of the three main channels inside the body; the characters seem to be trying to tell us that our brain is like an antenna that can connect with the universe.

### DEFINING SOUL IN CHINESE

Soul in English is represented by two words in Chinese, *ling hun*—spiritual soul. When referring to inspiration or brainwave, *ling gan*—the feeling from the spirit—is used. Many idioms expressing feelings are related to soul/spirit. When a Chinese person is scared, he says, "Oh, you almost scared my soul out of me!" To mean someone is scared out of his wits, the saying is, "It is as if the soul has left his body." When describing someone deeply disturbed, it is, "His xin and hun (heart-mind and spirit) are in an unstable state." If one is deeply in love and infatuated, the idiom is, "His *shen hun* (spirit and soul) are reversed." If someone has developed what we call intuition in the West, in qigong terms, intuition is related to the person's soul and spirit. The young Grand Master Xu Ming-Tang calls such explored abilities extrasensory abilities.

## Intuition

### INTUITION (SHEN TONG) AND HEART-MIND (XIN)

In different cultures, there are people who have revealed their potentials, or what is called intuition; this potential can be much more than just intuition. Several scientific researchers think that the diencephalon, also known as the interbrain, can function to keep a person young. According to many ancient and several modern qigong masters, when the governing qi channel (back along the spine) to the diencephalon is totally opened up, the person's third eye opens leading to one type of extrasensory ability. These people have acquired the ability to see and scan things that ordinary people cannot. Third eyes can open at different levels. According to the theories of Daoism, Buddhism, and qigong, such ability is only connected to her spirit, but yet not the spirit itself that is being revealed. In another words, the extrasensory ability is not the spirit itself, not the spirit shown in the person as defined in the Western term "enlightened." It is the same as those masters who are able to send their souls to do tasks for them.

Gaining extrasensory abilities is only part of the process of completing the journey to find the root of life and return to the origin, in other words, to achieve the ultimate attainment. We must understand that gaining these powers cannot prevent practitioners from becoming ill, aging, and dying. That is, if you want to pursue Dao, you must continue cultivating with diligence and sincerity. After having attained the status of an immortal/celestial, sickness does not occur in a master because her body has changed to beyond a regular person's bodily condition, which is "designed" to live on the earth. If such a master becomes ill, he can control his illness with his will. This is a different subject that is related to previous lives. You can find stories about this in my book, *Qi, The Treasure and Power of Your Body*.

I met a highly respected well-known Daoist, 100-year-old Zhen Yangzi who explained, "A baby has not lost his pre-birth (primary) qi, nor has the baby used their afterbirth xin (heart-mind). An older person can cleanse the stains and dirt [of the xin, spiritually] without losing the primary qi and scan widely and broadly both the ancient and modern world." What he is really talking about is the reason why it is easier for young children to reveal potentials when they practice qigong, and the potentials of knowing the truth of his life. The state of a baby's mind is the qigong state of mind when a master uses his extrasensory abilities. Such a state of heart-mind is also often the same as a high-level qigong master's.

The stories of the people who have extrasensory abilities may help explain how a person's xin (heart-mind) can coordinate with her spirit and demonstrate phenomenal performances. Such explored abilities however, are either in or beyond the so-called sixth sense. The term, sixth sense, in qigong practice is defined and functions differently than the way it is in the West. An extrasensory ability can be realized in a person who has some inborn special quality that has been revealed for some reason, or to sensitive people after they have practiced qigong for a long time and have reached a certain level. Some people have revealed their extrasensory abilities accidentally as did Master Ou and Master Wu.

### SHEN TONG, AND LONG CULTIVATION AND PRACTICE

High-level extrasensory abilities can occur only in a very special individual after many years of consistent cultivation and qigong practice. Extrasensory ability in Chinese is called *shen tong*. *Shen* means spirit or celestial and *tong* means to connect. *Shen tong* means to connect to the inner being of one's self. When you reverse these two words, they tell us where a person's extrasensory ability comes from—from the person's own inner being. Shen tong also means the abilities that lie beyond sensory abilities that can be explored at different levels such as the lower level shen tong called intuition in Western terms. I have met several qigong masters whose shen tong were at different levels. Some can "see" through subjects like a wall; others can scan only a vague picture, and yet others can scan more clearly and see much further such as finding out what I was doing from the other side of the globe. Some can read other people's thoughts vaguely, others can read the thoughts exactly. Some can move subjects around.

"All high levels of shen tong can only come from cultivation and deep chan meditation practice and also the accumulated achievements from previous lives." said the well-known Tibetan Living Buddha, Rinpoche Luosangtudanpai who added that, "Shen tong is only the method for helping people, not the goal of practicing. Only the shen tongs that rise above the conditions of the earth represent the real type of Buddhism." This teaching is identical in Daoism. He further emphasized in one of his books that, "Especially during this decade. Buddhist practitioners need to be alert about the false masters such as Falun Gong's founder, Li Hong-Zhi who in fact is not well-educated about Buddhism, but claimed himself to be the reborn-Buddha. There has never been a Buddha who claimed himself to be a reincarnation of a Buddha without being named by the people because of his life achievements. The consequences of such deception can be severe..." As you can see now, if the practitioner fails to cleanse the heart-mind or remains superstitious because of not knowing enough about qigong theory, unfortunate events can occur during prolonged meditation, especially if the practitioner is interested only in a narrow goal such as opening the third eye and personal gains. However, Daoism teaches us that one must keep the back door open so that the wrongdoer can have another chance and Buddhism teaches us that a wrongdoer can achieve salvation one he gives up evil doings.

Almost all the masters who have attained Dao hide their identities and their highly achieved shen tong. Achieving shen tong does not necessarily that a person has attained Dao—to be enlightened in the sense it is meant in the West. To have gained some shen tong can hasten the pursuit of Dao if the practitioner is wise. According to qigong theory, high-level practice means that one works on revealing one's own inner being, not focusing on gaining intuition.

## How the Inner Being is Revealed

### Ridding Oneself of the Yin-Devil

My research in ancient and modern high-level masters indicates that to reveal one's own inner being can only happen through meditation, yet meditation should not be the sole practice. To gain good health, the practitioner needs persistence, will, wisdom, caution, courage, and cultivation, as well as practice with moving forms. Besides all of these, the practitioner needs the freedom of time and the help of an authentic and good teacher.

The crucial part of working on the inner being is getting rid of the "yin devil." The yin devil represents the unseen negative energy that comes mainly from one's own mind. To ordinary qigong practitioners, if they do not cultivate and work on becoming big-hearted, the uncleanliness of the negative energy in the practitioner's subconscious can become the so-called yin devil. It is called "devil" because whenever there is a chance, this negative power will come out to disturb the practitioner's feelings. As a result, unhealthy feelings will harm the qi circulation and cause health problems for the practitioner. More seriously, in a prolonged meditation that extends for many hours, the yin-devil can even change a weak-minded practitioner's personality. The practitioner can become excessively delusional in matters of love and fear, lose consciousness, harm himself physically, become obsessed with someone, or become delusional about gaining extrasensory abilities. There have been some unfortunate incidences like these in China. When a qigong master has not cleansed his heart-mind adequately during prolonged meditation, the master cannot pass the test of the yin-devil and can become deluded.

Some of my personal experiences with ridding myself of the yin-devil, which is not an easy task, were described in my *A Woman's Qigong Guide*. If I am able to clear away the yin-devil that disturbs my carefree state of mind, I continue my meditation. If I fail to do this, I end my meditation immediately and stand up. I would rather be a healthy qigong practitioner than to become deluded on the path of my spiritual practice, realizing that in this lifetime I might not be able to become an immortal.

## MORAL CULTIVATION

For a practitioner pursuing high levels, all types of qigong practices demand moral cultivation. Cultivation is a "qigong lifestyle" that is described in my *A Woman's Qigong Guide*. Instead, here I want to focus on the most important part of cultivation—morality, which is the essential, crucial demand made on practitioners, especially at high-level practices. Interestingly, to emphasize good virtue is one way qigong is harmonized with the teachings of Western religions. Yet there are fundamental differences.

Qigong practice of any type emphasizes individual efforts, supplies different forms to suit different individuals, and emphasizes balance in physical health and in the mind. In another words, the individual is the sole "sponsor" or her spiritual practices in exploring her potential and becoming an immortal. The principle in all types of qigong is that a person's fate is in one's own hands, no matter if the practice is Daoist or Buddhist. Studying Daoism and Buddhism can increase one's ability to discover the true yin devil, true Daoism, and true Buddhism. When an immortal or a very high-level master chooses a student who has the potential to practice and eventually become an immortal, the master will demand good morality.

All the sages emphasized yin moral cultivation, regardless of which theory of immortality or Buddhist theory they espoused. Without working on yin morality, all say that no matter how high a level the qigong practitioner achieves, there is no way for him to attain immortality. Yin morality is even more important than yang morality in high-level qigong practice. Yang morality means the known, seen good deeds that the practitioner has done. The yin morality, on the contrary, is the unknown. Many sages wrote about and taught their students how to work on moral cultivation.

## Six Sticky Glue Balls

I have translated the Buddha's metaphor comparing our senses to the "six sticky glue balls," from the Buddhist classic, *The Da Yi*. The senses are hearing, seeing, taste, smell, feeling, and the mind. The classic says that our six sticky balls become larger and larger over the years, and then they gradually cover our own spirit light. In a young child, his six sticky balls are, of course, much smaller than those of an adult. Spiritually, young children are considered to be purer and closer to their own inner beings—their spirits. This is why it is easier for a child to reveal extrasensory abilities when practicing qigong. The Lord Buddha described our inner being as

> the round, glowing light that each person was born
> with...When one of the six sticky balls is pulled off, the
> practitioner will be able to catch a glimpse of his own
> spiritual light [that is, to attain Dao at a beginning lev-
> el]....He will then be able to continue working on getting rid
> off the rest of the sticky balls.

When pulling off the first sticky ball, starting from whichever ball works for you—the hearing one, the vision one, the mind one—you can become healthier and possibly gain some extrasensory abilities. To practice qigong and cultivate is a process of pulling off these sticky balls. There are practices designed for higher levels that can help you continue removing your six sticky balls, and explore more abilities at the yin spirit level

A good understanding of such gains is very important for the practitioner when advancing their practice. Without a thorough understanding of how and why have gained such abilities, practitioners will never have the chance to reveal their own spirits.

After much diligent practice and cultivation, the next level involves exploring yang spirits. Practitioners at this level no longer belong to the yin world where ordinary people's souls go after they die. They are in total control of their spirits, even of their physical bodies. They have become immortals, and even Buddhas. They have the freedom to either choose to stay in our yang world or move to different realms according to their abilities.

To remove the six sticky balls, you must make them smaller. In real life, when there is an emotional disturbance, one of the sticky balls expands. It then becomes more difficult for practitioners to improve their health, let alone continue the spiritual pursuit. Any disruptive emotions such as anxiety, greed, hate, sadness, lack of forgivingness, or excessive love can all make the six sticky balls grow larger. In Daoist terms, there is a drain on her own qi. Any emotional disturbances can interrupt the practitioner from accumulating qi and getting in touch with his inner being. In my own experience, even a tiny bit of emotion can unconsciously set up a battleground in meditation and interrupt the qi healer within. Willingly or not, the bit of emotion can fight off the qi healer's work.

The qi healer is able to work only when the mind has the freedom and authority to work on removing the blockages that cause health problems. In other words, only when the mind is totally peaceful and at ease (that is, relaxed and carefree), can the qi circulate well. After the qi healer fixes the health problem, it then works on prolonging the life span. In Daoist terms, to become strong and healthy is to learn how to nourish your own primary qi, "like a mother protecting the fetus," and to absorb qi from the natural world.

To make the process of removing the six sticky balls go more quickly, the practitioner must study, learn, and question with a clear, honest heart so learning becomes meaningful and helpful. My personal experience and research has taught me to grow in understanding Dao. This understanding includes what I may lose and what I have gained by just one careless thought; why the qi movements that made me feel good were just a beginning; why it seemed as if I was not making progress in my practice, but in fact I was; and how to handle things that happen during meditation. I have learned that to cultivate to reach simplicity is the way, but not the only way, and why simplicity is in fact the hardest to achieve. I have learned to continue working on purifying the heart (the yin morality) and being aware of constant disturbances because I am still human. I am continuing to cleanse the emotional disturbances, trying to be more tolerant, to practice persistently, so I can eventually "wash off" all the toxins caused by life.

No matter which goal you have, by walking on the qigong path, you can be certain of gains; you will have better physical and moral health. The fact of millions of people benefiting from qigong practice means that they can enjoy peace and a better life. In my book, *A Women's Qigong Guide*, I explained the underlying Chinese medical theory such as how qigong practice can effectively build up the inner organs.

I want to borrow Dr. Nan Hui-Jin's words to describe moral character,

> *In Daoist terms, human beings are like insects living on the plant Earth. Many of the ideas about space come from guesses, or are created in our own minds, or from what we think we know. The truth is, space is yet small. There is no way to know about it except practicing (qigong).*

How does one remove the six sticky balls? Having faith, I think, is the best way. In the process of removing the six sticky balls, you will feel yourself grow spiritually, as in the Chinese idiom, "grown like the beautiful lotus flower emerging from putrid mud." This saying is a favorite metaphor that many sages use. In *Nei Pian*, written by Bao Puzi (283–363 AD), a Daoist master and an expert in Daoist alchemy, says,

> *The parents are the "carriers", imparting qi and blood, and thus our bodies are formed. But, no one can tame a person's nature that a person is born with, yet a person can control her life by either cultivating, or going the opposite way. The Heaven cannot force anyone. A sage might die at an early age; a criminal person might live a long life. If Heaven has control, it may be the opposite.*

What he means is that our fate is in our own hands. To remove the six sticky balls is a self-effort practice and cultivation. Again, let me explain using Chinese terms. "To practice" in Chinese is called *xiu lian*—to exercise to adjust and refine. "To cultivate" is called *xiu xing*—to cultivate the behaviors and correct the wrong doings to retain nature. Specifically how can a qigong practitioner peel off the six sticky balls? The sages teach that becoming physically healthy and working on the heart-mind is the way.

As I wrote earlier, the celestials and Buddhas were those human beings who explored their potentials to very high levels. Now the question is: Where do we come from and where are we going at the ends of our lives. If Buddhas and celestials can emerge from us ordinary mortals by self-practice and cultivation, why cannot we see them around us? Why cannot we all explore our potentials as they have? How can we explore our Buddha seed? I've tried to provide some answers by digging into the sages' books, learning from high-level masters, and my own experience.

# CHAPTER 6

# Qigong Phenomena

## Introduction

Why are some qigong practitioners able to scan people's bodies even more accurately than the best machines? Such unbelievable phenomena are among the topics I am going to introduce in this chapter. First, I will tell you the story of a famous character—the "Monkey King" known by all Chinese in a classic novel written several hundred years ago. The novel's title is *Xi You Ji* (*Travel Notes Towards the West*). Nobody knows the real name of this author except for his pen name, Wu Chen-En. The true story of the Monkey King, named Sun Wu Kong (whose name means "the younger generation awakened by the void"), tells how he and other disciples helped Monk Tang (a true great master in Chinese history) to go to the West Heaven (where the Buddha lives) to fetch the essential Buddhist books. Although he has a monkey's head, the Monkey King has a human body and human characteristics. The stories in this novel, which have fascinated the young and old, tell how the Monkey King defeated or tamed devils and helped people.

During my visits in 1990 and 2000 to the White Cloud Monastery, the Vice Abbot Li Yu-Lin and the well-known Daoist Zhen Yangzi told me that both were quite sure this novel was actually written by Immortal Qiu Chu-Ji, the founder of the Daoist Dragon Gate School. After my ten years extensive research on qigong, I have come to realize that this novel indeed is a book about high-level qigong practice. The novel narrates how a qigong practitioner practiced and overcame his own inner demons to become a Buddha. The interesting stories describe the process and progress made in his high-level qigong practice.

The stunning powers and abilities of these celestials and Buddhas are described as "When qi forms into a shape, it forms a life; when qi scatters, it is invisible." Their bodies have become changeable (such as changing themselves into two or many, or into a different person or an animal). Such masters can have total control of their physical bodies and their spirits have been exercised and refined in ways beyond the understanding of ordinary people. In Buddhist terms, the levels that the immortals, celestials, and Buddhas achieved are the so-called seventh sense and eighth sense— terms that are unknown in modern science.

In this chapter, you will read several stories about real people who have revealed their potentials in different ways. Remember that to have gained some extrasensory abilities or even a high level of power does not necessarily mean that this person has attained Dao. My purpose in introducing these phenomena is to help you understand the potentials that human beings can reveal. I do not necessarily encourage people to seek such abilities. I must warn you that if a person practices qigong eagerly only to gain such abilities, the practice can only cause health problems, even to the point of mental illness. Such a selfish eagerness can cause qi to become tangled and create blockages in the qi channels; diseases then occur. Without learning enough and cultivating constantly, practitioners will not be able to solve such problems caused by tangled qi, nor can they handle the physical changes when the qi is cleaning and processing the body. Also, without high-level, experienced qigong teachers who have explored their own extrasensory abilities and can guide children, parents should not encourage their young children to practice meditation for just the purpose of revealing their extrasensory abilities. In my earlier book, *A Woman's Qigong Guide*, I also talk about children.

The many human potentials that qigong can explore, besides healing, are phenomenal, beyond what we see and know in life. This is why many people find it difficult to believe these phenomena, even during ancient times. Ancient people would become superstitious about a phenomenal incident that appeared once and worship it. Several times, emperors or officials in Chinese history even executed some qigong masters who demonstrated their stunning powers. One classic example recorded in the ancient Buddhist book, *The Essential Kenole Fa of Chan Mi*, describes what happened when the Lord Buddha showed his large, strong aura. Five hundred monks and nuns withdrew from his instruction because they were frightened and thought his aura was witchcraft. To this day, most exceptional masters hide their identities.

If you realize that phenomenal manifestations are only human potentials that can be explored through qigong practice, you will understand the science behind the phenomena described later in this chapter. Many phenomenal performances have been witnessed by millions of Chinese people, myself included. When I was a child, I watched a large person standing on an uncooked egg or on an empty matchbox without breaking it or crushing its contents. One qigong master did pull ups on a piece of paper and pulled his body over an electric light pipe like a gymnast. His body had become very light so that the paper and the glass pipe were not broken. I watched a master put a red-burning iron stick on his tongue and saw the saliva changing into steam. I heard the sizzling sound from his tongue, a scary experience. Amazingly, he was unhurt. I tried hard to pull the heavy sledgehammer that a master asked an audience member to use to hammer on his head. I read in the classic books about qigong masters walking on the surface of water or staying under the water for a long time without using oxygen.

Not long ago, I read an article written in the magazine, *Qigong & Science* (12, 1998), about a young qigong master who could hold his breath for a long time. Qigong Master Hu, who did this experiment with researchers, stayed under the water for 40 minutes. Chinese government leaders, science researchers, and journalists watched his performance. A qigong demonstration taped by Bill Moyer in Beijing also showed phenomenal human power. A group of young men, including an American student, pushed a 70 year-old qigong master down. At the end, these young men all fell to the ground by this old master's gentle pushing. In the movie, *Crouching Tiger, Hidden Dragon*, martial arts masters performed some qigong skills too.

All such demonstrations, including moving a subject or bending a fork with the mind, are called qigong skills, which are in some ways mind skills. According to qigong theory, all such qigong skills or extrasensory abilities, are revealed human potentials. Such demonstrations have shown us that the extrasensory abilities are not fabricated, nor hocus-pocus, but indeed need to be researched and studied. The phenomena constitute a complicated and mysterious field waiting for scientists to look at more closely. How powerful can a human being's power be? I say that there is no limit for exploration.

In Daoist terms, all qigong skills and phenomena are related to the role of qi. Before I tell you about the phenomena of *pi gu*, human aura, rainbow aura, and natural mummies in the sections that follow, I present some modern-day manifestations of the phenomena whose descriptions I have summarized from the Chinese magazine, *Qigong & Science* and from the *Shaolin Kungfu Photo Book*.

## Manifestations of Qi Power

### SHAOLIN MONKS

The performances by the Shaolin monks that people often dismiss as being only for show reveal that qigong practice can make even a man's delicate private parts stronger. In the book, *Shaolin Kungfu Photo Book*, journalists Liu Wen-Min and his colleagues published photos of the monks from the Shaolin Monastery demonstrating many difficult physical feats such as hanging a rock (over 25 kilograms) from a young monk's testicles and another of a monk pulling a heavy stone cylinder (over 250 kilograms) with his penis over some distance. Other photographs of Shaolin monks who demonstrated different qigong phenomena appear in the photo book, which also describes Buddhist, Chan (Zen) practice, and the Shaolin martial arts. The qigong elements of self-defense Shaolin martial arts have been well-known since the Tang Dynasty (618–907AD).

### A SILK EMBROIDERY

An archaeologist, Tong Zun-Jie helped to excavate the Ma Wang Dui Tomb in 1973 from the Han Dynasty (206 BC–220 AD). Among the thousands of valuable discoveries, a silk picture caught his eye at once. Tong, who practiced qigong, had a hunch that this silk embroidery picture was qigong guidance. He had an exact copy of it made and started to study it.

The 44 lifelike figures in the silk embroidery are shown doing various kinds of qigong movements; only 20 of the pictures include names and 13 have the names of the diseases these movements treated. The rest of the pictures look like a form, but with no accom-

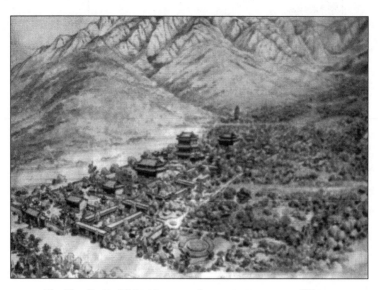

*The Shaolin Buddhist Monastery has over 1,470 years of history.*

panying instructions. Tong decided to imitate and practice those movements. Day after day, he learned to practice them to the point where he often forgot to eat. He practiced and practiced. One day, he suddenly felt as if he had entered an integral whole, and all those figures jumped off the pictures and joined him in his practice. Tong automatically followed their movements and soon felt a warm flow suddenly streaming out of his Shen Que point (an acupoint just inside the navel) into his Tian Mu point (the third-eye area). After a while, he ended the form, and found himself sweaty; he was alone—all those figures were still in the picture! He chuckled at himself and went to the kitchen where he found his wife sleeping soundly on the table. He woke her up and asked, "How come you are sleeping during the daytime?" His wife said, "I do not know." The same thing kept happening whenever Tong exercised—his wife fell sound asleep. Suddenly, Tong realized that this type of qigong was a hypnotizing qigong and he named this qigong Ma Wang Dui Guide Hypnotize Qigong.

In April 1986, he demonstrated the qigong form in the Beijing Capital Stadium in front of audience of thousands that included many highly positioned leaders. Over forty volunteers went on the stage, among them were medical doctors, Traditional Chinese Medicine doctors, the host of the Central TV Station of the government, and several doctrinaire Communist leaders including a military general who was ready to convince the public that this was all witchcraft. Tong began practicing and the general who tried hard not to fall asleep was one of the first people who fell into a deep sleep. One by one, all of the volunteers fell down and slept. One of them slept right next to the microphone; his loud snore made people laugh. When they were awakened up, some said their pain was gone and others said they felt very energetic. Tong went on to establish the Ma Wang Dui Qigong College.

### THOUGHT TRANSMITTANCE

The vice president of the Chinese Humanities Research Institute, Wang You-Cheng demonstrated qigong in 1991 before a group of overseas Chinese. For example, he put a coin on his Shan Zhong point (between the two nipples) and moved the coin with his mind; the coin moved 2 cm to the left. Next, he put two coins on his chest and used his mind to make the two coins move in opposite directions. During the demonstration, he also successively read the thoughts of other people and transmitted his own thoughts to a volunteer who was in another part of the city. The volunteer was a Chinese tourist from a south Asian country whom he had never met before.

During a second demonstration in Hong Kong that year, Master Wang was examined by Professor Wen-Jie Zheng of University in California at Berkeley, the vice chairman of Hong Kong Science Association, Professor Yu Zhao-Xun of Hong Kong University, and many other scientists and journalists. Professor Zheng went to another room and wrote down three things he had thought and put the note in his pocket. After he returned, he sat down in front of Wang. Wang told the audience what Zheng had written. Zheng took his note out of his pocket and showed the witnesses that Wang was correct. During that meeting, Wang also helped some of the audience in the front seats gain some extrasensory abilities. Ten days later, Master Wang did several experiments for several Canton City leaders where he read the thoughts of three leaders accurately. Wang explained to the journalists that,

> *Human beings' thoughts can cross over to the other side.*
> *Your left brain guides the right side of your body, the right*

*brain gives orders to the left side of your body, and the brain
can work on two different kinds of things at the same time,
such as when someone is playing a piano, or driving a car.
In some ways, what I did is similar toe a satellite that
passes pictures through a television from one side of the
earth to the other side. Because the qigong masters use their
power to pass their thoughts, their energy is different from
the satellite's energy. The picture from a qigong master
contains some qi energy; the qi energy can last and stay.*

Master Wang's story sounds unbelievable, doesn't it? But you will read about even more mysteries now.

### DEGENERATIVE BONE DISEASE

Mrs. Mai Yan-Qiong has become a well-known qigong healer and doctor in Hong Kong today. Several years ago, she suffered from what was diagnosed as a terminal illness. She had several extensive operations and could only lie in bed. The disease calcified her muscles and bones to the point where she became like a living mummy for two years. A friend taught her a quiet qigong form that helped her to focus the mind on breathing. She practiced the form persistently despite intolerable pain until her condition improved. Gradually she cured herself and became well. Afterwards, she learned more about qigong and studied at the Chinese Traditional Medicine University in Canton. She traveled throughout China and learned different types of qigong from many qigong masters. In addition to hosting a television program about qigong in Hong Kong, she established the Natural Healing Research Institute and a hospital in Hong Kong.

### THE MASTER'S TAPES AND QI ENERGY HARMONY

Do you believe that just playing audio or videotapes can help form a qi-energy field? Here is a report from the Xinjiang province where in 1990, Xin Jing Normal University and several other institutes jointly organized the Athletic Science and Qigong Conference. Eighteen meetings were held and 2,303 people of all ages attended. The audience included representatives from several minority nations and people from various professions. Of these, 1355 people came for treatments. They had different diseases such as arteriosclerosis, heart diseases, high or low blood pressure, and paralysis. Twenty-three people came to learn how to treat their family members' diseases because the family members could not come. Other participants came to learn more about qigong. In the hall, there were doctors and qigong masters standing on the sides in case anyone needed help; they also guided and corrected people's postures when Dr. Yan Xin's tape was playing. Before playing the tape, the doctors described qigong and Dr. Yan Xin's background. Afterwards, they taught his methods to the participants. The people started by listening to Dr. Yan Xin's tape and followed his instructions. The hall gradually formed a strong qi-energy field, and many people started moving spontaneously. After the public meeting ended, people were asked to continue doing this type of qigong an hour everyday.

According to the follow-up report, 80% of the audience paid close attention and followed the steps described in the tapes. A third of the patients showed obvious reactions in the areas of their illnesses of differing degrees, some reactions lasted a few minutes, some even lasted for hours at different times. Most of the reactions yielded good results. Another third of the patients showed reactions a few hours after the meeting, or even after one to three days. The reports showed that different individuals had different reactions and the reactions lasted from one to four days, after which the reactions disappeared. Nine hundred and eighty-five people had various kinds of spontaneous movements for ten minutes to even two and half hours. The longest lasted until the meeting was over.

After the thirteenth meeting, the researchers surveyed 985 people. They found that their spontaneous movements all related to the Chinese Five Elements Theory according to their own health problems. For instance, people who had stomach problem or neurasthenia would lie on the ground and roll around, or went to the wall touched the dirt. Such illnesses are related to the "Earth" element—the symbol of the spleen and stomach. People who had liver and gallbladder problems would touch wood—the symbol of liver. People who had breathing problems would breathe heavily like the roar of a tiger; people who had heart diseases would stretch arms like birds flying, and so forth.

The report added that after the conference, a third of the patients felt immediate health benefits; one third felt benefits after two to ten days; and a third felt that they did not benefit from the conference. Some of the reasons that these people did not benefit were they did not follow the steps and end the form correctly; they did not have faith in qigong so that they passed a negative message to their own bodies which had affected the healing (except when a high-powered master "aimed at" this person to give qi treatment). Among those who came to the meetings for their family members, 13 of the 23 family members made improvements.

All who attended the meetings reported that their memories improved and felt more energetic. Three people gained some extrasensory abilities such as scanning people's bodies. Eight began on pi gu; they stopped eating food but absorbed qi for three to twenty-one days. Unfortunately, they were all disrupted by their families and forced to stop being on pi gu because their not eating worried their family members. Three deaf children, ages 8, 11, 13, all

---

### Dr. Yan Xin's Life Story

After Dr. Yan Xin became famous in China, journalists interviewed people who knew him. Some of his colleagues said they had never seen anything unusual about Yan Xin, "He is just as ordinary as each of us!" But few told some amazing stories, including Yan Xin's family members, his wife, and his baby brother. All of the stories will be mysterious to you.

Dr. Yan Xin's former boss, one of the heads of the Mian Yang Traditional Chinese Medicine College witnessed Yan Xin's power when he was riding in a bus during a business trip with Yan Xin. He saw two thieves who simply could not pull out the wallets of a few passengers' pockets where they had put their hands in while Yan Xin was staring at them. The thieves kept saying, "I have seen some weird things today!" They looked around, and saw Yan Xin's eyes staring at them. They knew they had met a high-powered master and quickly got off the bus in fear.

Yan Xin's younger brother was spoiled when he was young; he feared nobody in the family except his oldest brother, Yan Xin. When Yan Xin was still living at home, his little bother sometimes caused trouble but never told his parents. But he could never fool Yan Xin because Yan Xin could read his mind; he would then be

recovered their hearing after one to five days. Six people had poor results that were caused by their leaving in the middle of the meeting, or not doing the end of the form. These six people went to hospitals where their doctors could not diagnose anything wrong. Later, they were treated by qigong masters for three to five minutes; their health problems were resolved. When the qi began to actively work on their health problems during a the meeting, these people suddenly stopped and left, thereby causing their qi flow to scatter. Their doctors could not find anything wrong because they said that hospital instruments that they had available could not scan the invisible energy movements.

## MOVING OTHER PEOPLES' BODIES

Can a high-level qigong master move your body around without actually putting a hand on you? An article in the *Qigong & Science*

---

punished for troubling other people. If he lied, Yan Xin did not even need to talk with him. If Yan Xin just looked at him, the young boy would be forced to remain in a standing posture, unable to talk or move for several hours. Yan Xin's wife said that Yan Xin's food supply for a whole month was only about one kilogram of peanuts and some water. He does not touch meat because he can see how the animal was butchered and this would make him sick to his stomach.

In the village in Sichuan where Yan Xin grew up, several stories have been widely told. One is about a thief who could not steal Yan Xin's parents' trees or cow any longer. The thief just simply forgot what he was doing when he went to steal grain and left what he had stolen behind. Dr. Yan Xin is a very caring son; no matter how busy he is, he goes home to see his parents on the Spring Festival. When people find out he is coming home, thousands of people wait for him. They call him "the living Buddha" because he has helped many people free of charge. Dr. Yan Xin says that he is just a human being and he cannot cure all diseases. Comparing his power with several people whom he knew, he said that his power was only a tip of a little finger! There are dozens of medical doctors now who have become his students and work for him in the United States.

magazine written by a Chinese journalist who followed a group of German students described their visit to a qigong master. In September 1988, a group of German students were watching qigong demonstrations in Zhe Jiang University. One of the performers was Qigong Master Chen Le-Tian's student. By using qi, he 'pushed' a German student who stood three feet away three meters further. Another student of Master Chen even used his qi energy to "push" two German students (who were standing behind the wall in another room) to walk a few steps. In another experiment, a master asked two students to stand back against and away from the wall. He used his qi energy to make one student walk towards the wall first until his head knocked the wall, while he was making the other student walk backward until her back was against the wall. All the German students deeply impressed by the demonstrations.

In July and August of 1993, Professor Cheng Hui-Xian, the former qigong instructor of the Oriental Medicine College of Oregon, took a group of qigong students to China. Those people saw some phenomena that they would never forget for the rest of their lives. In one of the demonstrations, a master from Tibet stood twenty feet away from a young girl and asked her to her close eyes. He used his qi energy to make her move her body left, then right, back and forth like a willow branch by just moving his fingers slightly. The girl felt her heart was being touched, and she sobbed. She felt her emotional pain, which had deeply rooted in her heart for years after a cruel incident, was being released along with her tears. Then she felt her heart being tickled, and she started to laugh and laugh until her pain was all gone. Ever since then, she has changed into a different person—I personally spoke with her.

Pi Gu at a Monastery

In the *Qigong & Science* (8, 1995), there is a photo of a 108-year-old female Daoist working in the field. The journalist who visited her wrote, "In Yu Xu Monastery, Wu Dang Mountains, there is a female Daoist named Li Cheng-Yu who became a Daoist disciple at the age of twenty seven and has lived in Yu Xu Monastery for 81 years...Although her skin is a little loose, it is smooth and fine. Her back is straight, and some of her white hair is turning black. A hospital that examined her found that she is very healthy; her pulse beats 72 times/min. She does not wear glasses, but can pull a thread through the eye of a needle. She sewed herself a patchwork coat made from many small pieces of fabric that she collected from tailor shops. Her teeth are so firm that she can bite hard nut shells as easily as children do. Her hearing is sharp, she moves quickly, and her body is pliable and strong. When she was 103 years old, she even had menses for three days and the color was bright red. Her life style is simple: meditate, live on *pi gu* regularly (not eating food but qi instead), and practice moving qigong forms. She needs only a very small amount of rice monthly."

In the following section, I will introduce more of what human beings can do. Please keep your mind open.

## What is Pi Gu

*Pi gu* means to live on qi, not eating food. Pi gu is, however, totally different from the fasting that is often practiced in the United States. Pi gu is a qigong practice during which the practitioners simply stop eating food, but eat qi instead. There are two types of pi gu practice. One is living completely on pi gu, which means the practitioners only "eat" qi without eating food at all, except some water. The other kind is the incomplete pi gu. People who practice the incomplete pi gu eat a little food, such as some thin rice soup and a little juice once in a while. Not everyone, however, is suitable and qualified to practice pi gu. Successful pi gu practice needs knowledge, the right conditions, and wisdom. In this book, I introduce this practice only to show you yet another method of developing the human potential.

Pi gu has been an important qigong practice in Chinese history. Over 7,000 years ago, qigong teachers taught the ancient emperor-sages the pi gu theory and practice. One of the earliest books, *Shan Hai Jing*, includes the story of a pi gu practitioner named Wu Guzi. The record described how he practiced pi gu, "He ate qi in spring when the sun rose, ate qi in autumn when the sun set, ate qi in winter at midnight, and ate qi in summer at noon—he followed the natural laws of yin and yang." In 1973, archeologists discovered fifteen Chinese medicine books in the Ma Wang Dui Tomb, some of which described qigong practices. One of the books described pi gu practice. The guidance given in this book tells how to start pi gu practice and explained that pi gu was an ancient practice of absorbing qi. The book written by Ke Heizi (between 586–618 AD) described pi gu practice, "The turtles can live without eating because of eating qi...After ten days of pi gu, you can eat some thin rice soup, or not eat food but still feel full because of eating qi." A book written by Bi Yan (618–907 AD) introduced his way of pi gu, "Absorb qi and then send it through the three channels...After 'eating' qi for fifty days, the grain in the stomach eaten before will be completely cleared out of the body. Then you can stop taking in anything, you can either eat a little food or without eating, both will become harmless. Your skin will look young and tender and smoother, and you can move more quickly."

Most masters who have been on pi gu for long periods do not want other people to know because the thought of not eating disturbs most people. There are several qigong practitioners who have been known to be able to absorb qi energy without eating for days, months, even for years. The Chinese magazine, *Qigong & Science* (1, 1994) published a photo taken by Mr. Kang, Jin-Yan early November 1993 (during the National Exploratory and Research Conference on Shi Hong-Qing in Ning Du county) of two female Daoists with a group of scientists, doctors, and journalists from different provinces and government agencies. Forty-nine researchers and several high-level qigong masters attended the conference. The purpose of the conference was to investigate the 25-year-old female Daoist Shi Hong Qing who had practiced pi gu for 1,027 days by the time the photo was taken. To the date of the photo, the female Daoist Shi Hong-Qing had not taken any substance except to drink a little water every few days. Nevertheless, she remained strong and healthy. Before becoming a Daoist in 1990, Hong studied with a 91-year-old woman qigong master. Before she passed away, her teacher told her to go into the monastery and become a Daoist. Now alone, Hong shaved her head and moved into the Qing Lian Monastery in Lian Hua Mountains where she still lives on pi gu.

The other female Daoist from the Jin Jing Dong Monastery is the 90-year-old Wen Si-Xian who is also famous for living on pi gu for many years. Wen eats only 2.2 pounds rice per month and her health is excellent. For over six decades, people in that area thought her as an ordinary Daoist. In 1987, Wen was invited by the county government to consult for the County History Museum program. Five young men went to fetch her because it was far from the monastery to the county museum, and there was no transportation in the mountains. All five had to walk. Surprisingly, they found that Wen, who then was eighty-four years old, could climb the hills much faster than them and not tire. During the three days of work, Wen ate nothing. Only then did people learn that Wen was a qigong master who had achieved a high level. The other eighty-seven year-old Daoist in Wen's monastery told the journalists that Wen stopped eating food over thirty years ago and only occasionally ate a little vegetable every few days, and a pound of rice each month.

During the ten-year Cultural Revolution, many monasteries were destroyed and the female Daoists lost their supplies. The Daoists in Wen's monastery started growing and selling vegetables to support themselves. Wen woke up every day at 3:30 in the morning and worked in the garden. She carried the vegetables in two baskets to the market at the foot of the mountain, which was over 6 miles away. After learning about her pi gu practice, a group of people sent by the government to visit Wen examined her and found that she was in good health, hears well, and does not even have presbyopia.

Both the two female Daoists and the other people who attended a conference who had been practicing some form of pi gu from different places were observed by the Academy of Somatic Science, the Qigong Research Institute, journalists and doctors for months. Their report on Shi Hong Qing was limited to the period during the 1027 days that she drank a little water only. Dr. Kang Cheng-Yan (M.D.) reported the test results on Hong from hospitals. Repeated tests indicated that there were mineral elements in Hong's urine and in her blood serum; their quantity was always normal. A professor from the Gan Nan Medical College reported the nutritional composition in Hong's body was normal and checked the microbial activity in her intestines. The experts, including high-level qigong masters, analyzed the data and concluded that because carbon, hydrogen, oxygen, and nitrogen existed in the air, Hong was able to absorb them into her body where they were changed into nutrition. Elements such as potassium, sodium, and calcium that do not exist in the air were found in Hong's body. If she does not eat food and only drinks a little water, where has she absorbed these elements? It is a mystery and a qigong phenomenon.

Others who were also on pi gu told their stories at the conference. Professor Liu Yu-Ping, a professor at Jiang Xi Province Teachers College, started on pi gu for 60 days. She felt more energetic and healthier during that period. In her later qigong practice, her pi gu spontaneously started a few more times. Another woman, Zhou Gui-Ling from Tian Jin City reported that she had suffered from hyperthyroidism and was about 44 pounds overweight. After practicing qigong, she cured herself, lost the extra weight, and then automatically began pi gi for sixty days. During that period, she started being able to scan other people's bodies and diagnose diseases. Now she can control when she goes on pi gu anytime she wants. Another member of Tian Jin City Somestic Research Institute, Wang Shu-Min reported how she suddenly began pi gu when she practiced qigong and gained extrasensory abilities.

PI GU AND CHILDREN

Some children are known to have been on pi gu as well as exhibiting extrasensory abilities after practicing qigong such as being able to scan people's bodies, and even being able to move subjects by their minds. Most of these children were not named in the literature in order to protect their privacy. To do pi gu as a child can, however, consume the qi and harm their health if done incorrectly. A group of researchers investigated a twelve-year-old boy for two weeks. This boy, who had been on pi gu for over two hundred days, never ate anything but once in a while drank some water during the period of observation. Nevertheless, he was healthy and stronger than before.

In 1992, the Military Medicine Research Institute followed a thirteen-year-old girl who practiced qigong and had stopped eating for thirty days between August 13th and September 12th. Doctors, journalists, and government representatives observed the young girl around the clock during the experiments. The hospital used Western and traditional Chinese methods during clinical examinations of the girl. There were 140 types of tests, including daily activity, blood, routine urinalysis, immunophysiology exam, electro-physiological exam, endocrine, routine examination, trophism, work physiology, mental quotient exam, and others. During the thirty days, the girl only drank 984ml water daily, and four times she drank small amounts of juice. Despite not eating food and being underweight, the girl's health was excellent. During the 30 days, she urinated four times with average daily amount of 656 ml, and had a bowel movement only once, 54 gm in weight. She lost approximately nine pounds, of which seven was fat. Blood tests showed that the hematochrome, red blood cells were normal, or slightly lower in the normal range. The serum test showed that all elements remained at normal levels, as was the TSH level. Her urine T3 determination thickness was reduced, her folliculinuria and estradiol was higher than most adults, and her estriol level was lower than normal.

## PI GU DURING SPACE SIMULATION

From May 1986 to January 1987, Qigong Master Zhang Rong-Tang used his Rotating Qigong at the Space Medical Science and Technology Institute in Beijing during space simulation experiments. He successfully made the highest score for astronauts, and he was already over fifty years old. He suggested a pi gu trial in a space simulation as a way to understand how qi worked in the universe, or maybe how extraterritorial beings might live. At the Zhe Jiang Province Chinese Traditional Medicine Hospital, he did a pi gu experiment. After 21 days' pi gu, his body's immune system increased, his health was not harmed, and his fat and blood lipids were clinically reduced.

## PI GU AS A MEDICAL TREATMENT

Pi gu is an important subject of scientific research in China. Supported by the local government and hospitals, Master Zhang Rong-Tang has set up many extensive pi gu workshops. He has also helped patients practice pi gu, that is, to learn qigong and absorb qi from the universe. He also founded a Pi Gu Hospital. The following are some case studies of his patients who learned to practice pi gu for treating their diseases.

A 45-year-old male patient was diagnosed with diabetes and hepatitis B at his former hospital in 1985. After he took medicine, his GPT (glutamic pyruvic transaminase) level rose. He had to stay at home. In April and June, he went to the Pi Gu Hospital twice to practice pi gu. His hemoglobin count turned from positive to negative, his GPT fell to 50U and soon became normal. His blood sugar decreased from 200 to 100mg/dl. Later after a few more periods of being on pi gu, his cholesterol decreased from 328 to 195mg/dl, triglycerides decreased from 556 to 72mg/dl, and his blood platelet count rose from 60 thousand to 110 thousand/mm3. He has recovered and is now working.

A 55-year-old female patient was told at the Hong Zhou Hospital that her cancer, a well-differentiated phosphorus cell cancer, had reached an advanced stage and that her condition did not allow her to have an operation. In May 1989, she went to the Pi Gu Hospital where she gained the ability to scan herself as if in an X-ray. As she practiced pi gu, she could see that the cancer was gradually becoming smaller and later disappearing. On June 7, hospital examinations did not find cancer cells. She has been well ever since.

In another 52-year-old female patient, the Canton Zhong Shang Hospital found a 16.2x11.9mm tumor in the left ventricle of the heart. She did not want an operation. Instead, in February 1993 she went to the Pi Gu Hospital where she practiced pi gu for twelve days for the first time. In the next month, her hospital found that her tumor was gone.

Master Zhang Rong-Tang pointed out that it is not necessarily better to do longer pi gu periods. For better results, do it periodically with pi gu masters as guides. The journalists who visited six people on pi gu in Su Zhou City found similar results: after doing pi gu for over ten days, every one of them lost some weight, but after a certain point, the weight loss stopped automatically at the weight that the person should according to their height. When they stopped eating food, they did not feel hungry or were uninterested in food except water. During that pi gu period, if they forced themselves to eat, they did not feel well. To be successful, they had to absorb qi every day, several times a day. They could absorb qi anywhere they wanted. To stand under pine or fir trees made them feel good. They said they could tell if the tree was sick—the qi would "taste" bitter.

Grand Master Want Zi-Shen's teacher, a well-known Tibetan Master Mong who just passed away several years ago had lived far away from the monasteries in the mountains. The Communist authorities locked up the teacher in the 1950s for no apparent reason. As a protest, he refused to eat any food for half a year, yet he remained healthy. The government set him free because it was afraid something would happen to him.

## Human Aura

Aura is light, but only in different shapes. According to qigong theory, human aura is qi. When a person glows, it is the yang qi. Chinese medicine doctors check the facial color for the qi "aura." When I was a young child, my aunt who liked to tell children's stories told us that each of us "had an aura." She said that our auras could scare a ghost away. I did not understand what she meant but believed her.

Chinese children often received an informal education on human energy from listening to adult conversation or going to special performances. When I was in grade school, I watched a well-known comedian's show in the theater. He said, "At midnight, if you walk through a graveyard, do not turn back quickly if you hear someone calling you, but turn slowly like this." He then turned very slowly in a rigid way, his whole body looking as stiff as a pole. He went on to explain, "so the lights on your shoulders won't be blown off and scare the ghost away." Pausing, he added, "But do not turn like this in the street. If in the street all people turn like this..." and he and his partner turned around like poles with the limbs rigid and stiff. As a child I thought it was funny and I laughed so hard until tears came to my eyes. But now I think his story told me something related to human aura.

When I was teaching high school in the 1970s in China, a colleague practiced qigong and treated people's diseases. In a dimly lit room, his hands gave off a dim pale blue light while he treated a patient.

In 1985, Professor Yang, a Chinese scholar from the Chinese Industrial University in Beijing who was visiting Oregon State University, used qigong to cool a young student's high fever after a hospital had failed to find the cause of his continuous high fever. While Yang was giving qi to treat the young man, his fingers gave off a dim pale blue light. In China, many people show their auras while doing qigong. When I went to China to visit my relatives and friends, some showed me photos that they took of the qigong practitioners who had auras above their heads. A strong aura like a beam of a flashlight could be seen on the head of Mr. Zhou who has practiced Soaring Crane qigong for over ten years.

Dr. Yan Xin, who has experimented with qigong phenomena,

explains that the visible human aura is the qi energy of a human being. According to qigong theory, aura is qi energy and each person's aura differs according to the practitioner's health. In an ordinary person, the more qi energy a person has, the stronger the aura will be. The aura does not necessarily mean this person has extrasensory abilities that a qigong practitioner has explored. The higher qigong level a person achieves, the stronger her aura is and her energy becomes available for treating diseases. More scientists and people have learned and realized that an aura—qi that comes from within ourselves—can be induced by qigong practice and reduced by poor health.

The auras on different qigong practitioner's heads are shaped differently. Some are round as around the heads of the sages. Their auras look different because they were at high levels. I have seen round auras shown in photos taken by Chinese journalists. For example, the Grand Fragrant Qigong Master, Tian Rei-Shen can emit his bright, big aura when he wanted to show people. His head aura resembled those of the sages or saints in Western churches. Master Tian showed his aura before several thousand people several times. He can show a bright aura around his body and his hands. Some of these photos taken by journalists are collected in his book, *The Fragrant Wisdom Qigong*. Grand Master of Zhong Yuan Qigong, Xu Ming-Tang showed strong auras in his three dan tians at the same time in a photograph taken by Ukraine scientists. In 1997, the previous president of the National Qigong Association in the United States, Dr. Russel Dematis showed two hundred attendees a photo of a young qigong master. There was a round circle of white aura emanating from his head, not too strong, but nevertheless clear.

## Rainbow Lights

Higher level qigong masters can choose to leave the earth without leaving behind any part of their bodies and suddenly disappear in colorful rainbow lights or just a few snow-white balls like the Lord Buddha did. In the early 1960s, the then communist Commander in Chief of Tibet, General Zhang Guo-Hua together with his colleagues witnessed this phenomenon in Tibet. An old monk notified an authority to come on the day when he decided to leave the earth. On that day, he sat on the ground in the open on a square with many

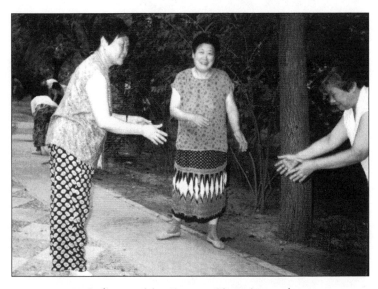

*Ladies practicing Fragrant Qigong in a park.*

people around him in a big circle. He sat and meditated, then, suddenly, a rainbow-like light formed—he had left our world.

A well-known Tibetan Buddhist-style qigong master, Wang Zi-Sheng, who has been to Tibet many times says that in the past forty years, there were thirteen monks in Tibet who passed away by disappearing in rainbow forms. Several such high-level masters wanted to leave something to the later generations such as the Lord Buddha did. The Buddha told his disciples to burn his body, and his cremated remains contained a few snow-white materials called *she li zi*. The Indian Buddhists gave a piece to the Chinese in ancient times. In the 1980s, this she li zi was found in a gold box hidden in a pagoda in the temple in Baihai Park, one of the former imperial parks in Beijing. There have been numerous high-level qigong masters in the entire country who left she li zi after their bodies were burned. Such material can be colored, too. According to Daoism, it is the jing of the masters that changes into visible material by the fire.

## Natural Mummies

Egyptian mummies are the ancient dead bodies that were processed with chemicals so the bodies could be preserved. In this section, I introduce you to "natural mummies," a term I use to describe the bodies of deceased high-level qigong masters that were self-preserved naturally without the help of others or chemicals. Masters who wanted to leave their bodies body forever on the earth because at the time of their death, their their qigong levels were not high enough to change their bodies into rainbow light or who could not fly away turned themselves into natural mummies. Without using any chemicals or being processed by other people, the qigong master's body does not decay, but will harden by itself or over time. Some dead bodies can remain "fresh" for a long time. These natural mummies never rot. According to records in monasteries, some masters also took certain herbal formulas to cleanse their bodies when preparing for death. They were all able predict their time of passing; they could prepare themselves and their bodies ahead of time. Depending on the levels that they had achieved, some could leave their bodies soft and elastic, and others could harden their bodies into statue-like states. The sizes of the hardened bodies depended upon the levels of these masters. The higher the level, the smaller the body became. The size could remain life size or shrink to be as small as the size of a hand's palm or a date. The higher gong they gained, the smaller they could shrink their bodies at the moment they passed away.

Grand Master Wang Zi-Shen told me that there are eleven such bodies in the Jiu-Hua Mount Monastery. When I went to Tibet in the summer of 2001, I also visited the Shigatse Monastery where most of the Panchans' bodies are kept. The Panchans, who are the Kings next to the Dalais, have been some of the main Tibetan Buddhist leaders. I was told that the body of a Panchan who died in the 1980s is still soft and grows hair.

In 1995, I heard on the radio that a small human statue was found in a cave in a North American mountain. A laboratory tested the statue and found that this statue had a complete organ system like a real human being. Could this statue be the body of an unknown high-level qigong master? If so, this discovery shows again how small our world is.

According to Li Wan-Xuan's survey (*Qigong & Science* 2, 1994), there are over ten qigong mummies now displayed in China. Some are over a thousand years old, some are several hundred years old, and some are just forty or fifty years old. One of the mummies was of Master Monk, Wu Ji of the Tang Dynasty who lived in the Nan Tai

Monastery in the Nan Heng Mountains, Hunan province. He passed away in 790 AD According to the monastery's records, a month before he died, Master Wu Ji told his disciples that he would pass away in a month. He stopped eating solid food and cooked herbal soups for himself to drink. On the specified day, he told his disciples that he was ready to go, but not to bury his body after he passed away. He sat quietly and meditated, and stopped breathing. One month after he died, his body began giving off a fragrant smell. His body has remained in good shape since then. His eyes are lifelike. His body was enshrined and worshipped in the monastery until the 1930s. A Japanese spy, by the name of Si Lang, went to the Nan Tai Monastery and pretended to study there. The monks took care of him, but Si Lang poisoned them and then shipped Wu Ji's body to Japan. Not too long ago, Si Lang died. Some Japanese people read Si Lang's diary and found out what he had done. They found Master Wu Ji's body hidden between the walls inside his house. Wu Ji's eyes were still lifelike.

A Taiwanese Master Monk, Tsi Hang, passed away on May, 6th, 1954. Five years later when his students opened the burial jar and checked his sitting body, they found that his body was still soft, his hair had grown on his head, and his eyebrows had become even thicker!

In February, 1985, a monk by the name of Da Xing passed away. He had lived in the Shuang Xi Monastery in the Jiu Hua Mountains of the An Hui province. His disciples kept his body in a big jar and buried him. After four years when they opened the jar and checked, a thick sandalwood fragrance wafted out and his body remained in the same state as when they put him in the jar.

In 1993, in the Hu Zhuang Zi village, Le Chang County, Canton province, a 79-year-old woman, Liu Yin-Zi, had been on pi gu since 1971; she ate only one meal every six days. Suddenly she told her family to prepare for her funeral. She told her family not to bury her body, but to keep it on her bed for scientific research. Four months later, a journalist who had visited her body after she died returned to see the body again. He saw that her body was still in the same shape although the summer weather there was hot and humid. Only her skin became a little dried with more wrinkles

An article in *Qigong & Science* written by Xiong Dan-Yu in 1994 described a similar case. An 88-year-old woman, Zhou Feng-Chen from Xiang He county in the He Bei province told her family suddenly to prepare for her death. She was a Buddhist and had practiced meditation for many years. She was also a vegetarian. The villagers said that she treated patients and had done so for free for many years. She told her grandchild that she knew when she would "leave." Before she died, she asked her family not to bury her body, but keep her body on the bed, also for scientific research. Journalists who visited the body over the past five years found it drier, but nevertheless in good condition.

Some interesting stories from a book written by Xu Xia-Ke who lived in the Ming Dynasty (1368–1644 AD) tell about qigong practices. Xu Xia-Ke spent most of his life traveling all over the country. His extensive research made an enormous contribution to geography as well as in unearthing local customs in Chinese history. Xu considered it important for a researcher to sincerely seek the truth from facts. As a qigong practitioner himself, Xu was not superstitious at all. He always criticized and clarified superstitious beliefs and unfounded qigong frauds and rumors. Between 1613 and 1639 AD, Xu Xia-Ke visited 382 monasteries, including 179 monks and Daoists. In his diary, he recorded what he had witnessed from those masters, such as their being able to show bright auras around their bodies and the fragrant smells given off by their bodies when they practiced qigong. He wrote that in the Lang Shi Monastery in Dao Zhao area in the Hunan province, there was the body of a Daoist who passed away several hundreds years before that was preserved in the monastery; its face was still soft as if he were alive. Xu described two other qigong mummies that he visited. One was the daughter of Li who was the governor of the Hunan province. The other body was a monk's from the previous dynasty—the Yuan Dynasty. Many more qigong phenomena are recorded in Xu Xia-Ke's book; indeed, he can be considered a great scientist in Chinese history.

# CHAPTER 7

# Qigong and Sexual Relationships

The English word "sex" means the sex of a person, male and female, or it means sexual activity. Both are considered important factors in qigong practice as well as in diagnoses and treatment in Traditional Chinese Medicine (TCM). In this chapter, I want to focus less on the sex of the female or male subjects because much of this information was included my earlier book, *A Woman's Qigong Guide*. Instead, I would like to focus on the sexual relationship between two people of the opposite sex.

## The Inferior Status of Women in Chinese Culture

Before going into detail about how qigong influences sexual relationships, I would like to touch on some negative aspects of the sexual culture in China. Simply put, men and women are treated differently, with women receiving the negative treatment. Even in Buddhist practice, a sample teaching says "To love a beautiful woman only ruins the physical body more quickly." I want to discuss how this negative attitude toward women evolved, because it is indeed related to qigong practice during history and in today's China. I think that when the status of the female began to be degraded in Chinese culture as well as in many other cultures in the world, this negative energy was the beginning of human beings degrading themselves. Even Buddhist nuns are called second-rank monks. To classify females as second class did not originate in Chinese thought. Tracing this negative attitude to women back in history, we find that in ancient Daoism and immortality practice, men and women were considered equally important because they were the yin and yang, and the heaven and the earth. These are ideas that still prevail in immortality practice and Daoist religion. From earlier classic novels, we can see that women's situation was much better before the Tang Dynasty. According to several Chinese scholars' research, it was after the Tang Dynasty (618–907 AD) that Chinese women started to be considered second class citizens. How did the belief that men are more important than women develop in Chinese culture? In this introduction, I attempt to give a background of this development. Please understand that I am not against men, nor do I think that men and women should compete for status. I am trying to simply untangle a snarled history, to trace the thread back to its beginnings.

The belief that a man must have a son was developed by a group of Confucian scholars during the Song Dynasty over one thousand years ago. Not having a son indicated a lack of filial piety and fraternal duty; it was a powerful belief that still strongly influences people, especially the farmers who do not have much education. In today's mainland China, some farmers still blame their wives for giving birth to girls. When I was a child, the women in the neighborhood often told me, "Be good, in the next life you'll be reborn a boy!" In old China, a rich man could marry many wives in order to have a son. Encouraged by the belief that men must have a son, men overshadowed women.

As in many cultures in the world, sex is a subject in Chinese culture that is still not discussed in public because of the sense of shame accompanying such talk. A Chinese husband could fulfill his "duty" with his wife without thinking much about enjoyment. The history and culture of China underlying these beliefs can be seen in the Chinese-American movie, *The Joy Luck Club*. The binding of feet at young ages by Chinese women is another example showing that women had become private property.

Over 500 years ago, a gifted Confucius scholar wrote lush pornography in his beautifully written novel, *Jin Ping Mei* (*The Plum In a Gold Vase*). In this novel, a man named Xi Men-Qing enjoyed sexual pleasure with several beautiful wives as well as with other women. The many pornographic drawings in this book might have included almost all the entire range of pornography in the world! This book also contains much information about how to build up a kidney's jing in the male by using herbal formulas and diets for longevity while enjoying sexual pleasure. At the end of the novel, the author had Xi die of excessive sexual pleasure an possessed with a wicked mind.

Only one woman in Chinese history ever ruled China the way several queens in the West did. During the Tang Dynasty, an emperor's wife seized power from her son when her husband died (around 650 AD). She named herself Wu Ze-Tian (*ze* means principle and *tian* means heaven). She became a powerful and capable Emperor (she was not called Empress) who ruled China successfully for many years. Although Wu Ze-Tian was powerful and achieved some economical reforms, historians always dismiss her, not only because she was female, but also because she did what many male emperors had done—enjoyed sex even though she kept her male lovers a secret. She did not keep many lovers inside the Forbidden City as a male Emperor might have, but had a few lovers early or later in secret. Still she was criticized as being lascivious. In Chinese history, if an emperor failed to produce a dynasty, the blame would often lie on the beautiful women that he loved.

There are women who are well known in history for supposedly ruining the country because they enjoyed sexual intercourse with their husbands. An empress during the Han Dynasty by the name Zhao Fei-Yan, who was also wonderful dancer, was blamed for the death of the emperor, because she and her sister used herbs to arouse the Emperor's sexual desire to the point he was died of surfeit. Both sisters were executed for this crime. Another well-known beauty, Yang Yu-Huan, who was the favorite concubine of the Tang Emperor Xuan Zong, was hanged when rebels took over the capital. She was blamed for having caused the Emperor to rule the country poorly and thereby causing rebellions. These women were called lascivious, guilty, and shameless. So-called lascivious women were cruelly punished during the Song Dynasty. If a woman was caught having an affair, she could be forced to ride on a donkey in a public parade with a long wooden stick poking inside her vagina. As you can see, the history that made women second-class citizens, sexual objects, and victims developed into a standard set of beliefs. Today, while women's situation in the West has improved much, most women in the world are still mired by old ways of thinking.

Women in China having acquired the status of second-class citizens affected them even in qigong practice. The taboo on talking about sex prevented the handing down of important and essential qigong practice teachings for women. Because of this history, most qigong books and diet books for longevity in China are written for men. Although men and women can share many qigong practices as well as diets for longevity. This contrasts to what ancient Chinese philosophy actually taught. As a result qigong theory has become distorted causing some misunderstanding of qigong. Qigong practitioners must recognize this distortion.

I personally think that in some ways, this ignorance in classifying women in Chinese history, consciously or unconsciously, originated from some well-respected scholar-masters who enjoyed high prestige, but misunderstood qigong practices. Lesser disciples of the real masters possibly handed down incorrect information. The result has been that ordinary qigong practitioners have not understood women's role since ancient times. Misunderstandings may have come about because of the female's physiology. It is true that in qigong practice, a female practitioner has to be concerned with her menses and pregnancy. In advanced practice, women have more parts than men to take care of. These differences, however, can also be "highways" that can speed up the female practitioner's progress— if the practitioner is taught by the right teacher who is knowledgeable and experienced. A practitioner can choose this "highway" or not based on her goals. In a Daoist practice designed by Immortal Lu Don-Bi during which a woman reached a higher level, the practitioner would eventually physically "look like a man" in some ways. Her menses might stop and even her breasts might change to those that look like men's, while the rest of her figure remains like a regular female's. She can regain her menses again if it is necessary. The practice is intended only to prepare for the more advanced practice, not for any other purpose. (I will include a few practices of this type in my next book on qigong for women.) In contrast to females, a male practitioner does not need to do extra work.

Possibly this extra work and the phenomenal physical changes into a "man-like" state in women's high-level qigong practice may have caused misunderstandings that were partly responsibility for the degradation of women's status. This division of men and women into two different social statuses merely on the basis of their physical difference probably originated with uninformed male practitioners. I say "uninformed." In the earliest Chinese books such as the *I Ching*, *Nei Jing*, and *Dao De Jing* which are the fountainheads of qigong,

Chinese medicine, and culture, I see nothing that is used to classify men and women separately. In fact, these books considered men and women to be equally important. These misunderstandings have become a part of Chinese culture. This is why I think that if the secret parts in qigong theory are clarified, the public can gain a better and deeper understanding of the true Chinese culture.

Next, I want to discuss the impact of modern thinking about sex on qigong practice. Sex, as a subject, has become very popular in many American television shows and movies. In many ways, the overtly sexy shows display much ignorance and also confuse many people, young and old. We often hear sayings like, "If you do not use it, you lose it!" "Experiments have proven that there is only sugar in semen." But are these sayings scientific? Are those researchers certain that that there is only sugar in semen as found in some laboratory results? Perhaps we should not close the door because the human body is far too complex and mysterious for modern science to completely understand yet? From other chapters, we learned about the different potentials we human beings can explore, but also that there have not been many scientists who study them and do experiments. Sex is an important issue in all cultures including Chinese culture. The philosophy of sex is, however, quite different in China than from the rest of the world.

## Defining Sex in Chinese

In qi culture, sex, *xing* in Chinese, is related to Chinese medicine, diet, longevity, and qigong practice. The sexes are also defined philosophically in ways that differ from the rest of the world. This difference can be found in the way the Chinese characters are written and used. For example, whereas the English word, "nature" refers to the natural world, it is two words in Chinese, *zi ran,* (自然) "naturally there." When "nature" is used in Chinese language to refer human beings, the word xing is used. The character, *xing* is formed by a "heart side" and "to produce." (性). Xing used in qigong terms means the "root of life." But when xing is used together with different words, different ideas are indicated such as sexual activity, different sex, or the personality one is born with. A person's natural temperament is called *xing ger* where *ger* means quality, standard, level. When using xing with *pin* ("to value,") it forms the term, *pin xing*, which refers to good or bad morality. Another example of the way many characters are written, is the character, to love, *ai* (愛). This character, love, is formed by the character "heart" placed together with "friend" under a roof with three dew drop-like dots. Any word that relates to human nature all have the "heart" or the heart side as part of this character. But none of the words that mean purely sexual pursuit such as having an affair, *tong jian* (通奸), to rape *qiang jian*, (奸), masturbate, *shou yin* (手淫) has this "heart" as part of these characters. Even the characters and terms that express excessive sex, *she yu*, (奢欲) show that such attitudes are not derived from human nature, but from the human mind.

Chinese characters show us in their written forms that some behaviors are foreign to human nature. From these characters, you can see that in Chinese culture, sexual behavior is related to nature originating from the heart and that sexual activity is an important part of our nature. Before you read the rest of this chapter, I would like to tell you that even many Chinese are confused about the word, jing. This misunderstanding is related to a misunderstanding about female qigong practice. The Daoist terms, jing (精), qi, and shen are well known, even in America. This word can mean either the "semen jing" in terms of Chinese Western medicine and the essential jing," which is related to qigong practice and Traditional Chinese Medicine. Not only some ordinary Chinese, but even some qigong practitioners who are not well informed are confused about the way the word jing is used differently. In Chinese medicine and qigong theory, both types of jing are produced by the kidneys. Yet they have totally different meanings in qigong theory and in medical terms that refer mainly to semen. In qigong theory, jing refers solely to the primary jing, which is directly related to the afterbirth jing that has much to do with semen. Remember, I did not say, "the semen" but said, "has much to do." Jing is a very complicated theory that I introduce only briefly because jing plays an important role in sexual relationships.

From this brief introduction you can see that there have been some misunderstandings about the terms, jing, qi and shen. Before you read further, I want to say that although I have taught many qigong classes and have done extensive research, I do not think I will ever teach a sex and qigong class. My little bit of experience resulting from my meditation has taught me that the similar sexual arousing sensation occurring during meditation is related to the essential jing. This bit of experience is enough to convince me the truth of what I have researched, studied, and learned. Now let us see how jing, qi, and shen were defined by the Daoist expert, Master Chen Ying-Ning. He emphasized,

> The top class types of practice all begin from the pre-birth qi [the primary qi] but not the afterbirth qi [the qi that breathes through the nose]. This theory has been written in all of the books from all of the different Daoist schools. The primary jing does not mean the jing from sexual inter- course; the primary qi does not mean the breathing qi. This is the important principle of Daoist practice that should be brought to people's attention.

Since I consider myself to be primarily a translator on the subject of this chapter, what I write here is mainly for reference and education; the material does not represent teachings from my own experience.

## Qigong and the Sexual Lives of Couples

For couples to have a moderate sex life has always been impor- tant in Chinese culture in that it is related to qigong practice and Chinese medical theory. The sexual arousal occurring in a relation- ship is related only to the heart-mind and belongs to the subject of longevity. The sensation that is similar to sexual arousal that hap- pens during meditation in any type of qigong practice—whether Daoist, Buddhist, or immortality—is not from the heart-mind, but from nature. This sensation arises from the movement of the qi itself when the practitioner is in the void state (xu). At this moment, the practitioner will feel as if he or she is aroused sexually, but this sensation is not totally the same as the arousal during intercourse.

This period, an important one for qigong practice, is called the live $zi$ hour to harvest the $yao$ (yao is the primary qi). The length of time of this sensation state lasts can differ, as can the periods of timing and the degrees. The sensation can appear and disappear in a matter of seconds, or it can last for a few minutes, hours, or even days, depend- ing on the ability and level of the practitioner. The moment for harvest- ing yao is named "the active live zi hour" in Daoist terms. $Zi$, which means hour, actually refers to earth time, the midnight hours between 12:00 A.M. and 2:00 A.M. Some use 11:00 P.M.–2:00 P.M. to include the time when the yang energy deep in the earth begins rising. When the term is used in qigong practice, it means the time when their yang energy (yao) begins to be active and is produced.

Many practitioners, ancient and modern, who have experienced the yang arousal state have described the sensation, which is a sensitive and crucial period in a qigong state. The practitioner can successfully handle and harvest the yao day after day, month after month, continuously. To harvest the yao without draining the essence is to build a foundation for further advanced practice, i.e., to harvest the dan, a process of reversing the biological body and pursuing immortality. If the practitioner is able to complete the process, that is, they are able to move beyond this whole period, they will then be able to move on to the next level in their qigong practice. This sensation of arousal occurs in all types of qigong practices, including the Southern Daoist and Northern Daoist schools.

According to Grand Master Nan Huai-Jin, some Tibetan Buddhist monk-masters can retain this continuous indescribable sensation period for twenty-one days. This naturally occurring sensation experienced mentally and physically is described as an incomparable pleasure, compared with sexual intercourse between a man or a woman. This pleasure increases as the practitioner continues his or her practice, to a level that the ancient Chinese practitioners described as "comparing this with the sex between a man and a woman, sex is like chewing a piece of tasteless wax. No one would want to trade this with the crown of an Emperor." In Buddhist terms, the master who has achieved this state is called the Happy Buddha. Ancient and contemporary qigong masters who have experienced such super pleasure all have said that this pleasure was beyond description. No other pleasure can compare with this pleasure that occurs in the meditation state. This sensation marks an important period for the practitioner to move to a higher level. After this period of training, the practitioner will increase her ability to face real life.

Many practitioners fail to move beyond this period. They remain stuck in this period, which means they cannot handle sensation and frequently would go to their women just to release their semen, thus regressing in their practice. If the practitioner releases his semen infrequently, his health and possibly his longevity, is not affected. It will be impossible, however, for this practitioner to pursue immortality. Many classic Chinese qigong books emphasize that when practitioners begin to experience this pleasure period and fail to handle it properly, all the efforts that they have made will be wasted; they will end up being ordinary persons. If the practitioner does learn how to handle this period and does not overindulge, the person would be able to continue to higher levels. I know practitioners who either have moved beyond this period or failed to do so. If the practitioner had not mastered the skills, but tried to hold his essence, health problems can arise. Only the wise, smart, and strong-willed ones can advance their practices. Many practitioners have succeeded in China. (Here we are talking about pursuing high-level qigong practice and, possibly, immortality, which is quite different from skillfulness in the bedroom and different from the sexual sensation aroused by the mind.) Another important difference between bedroom skills and immortality practice lies the goals. Bedroom skills help people have a healthy long life. The immortality practice is done to ensure longevity so that the practitioner has enough time to reach her final destination.

My qigong practice experience and learning has convinced me that our bodies can be changed by qigong practice in ways that modern science can only partly explain. There is much that remains opaque to modern science. I have studied many branches of the different qigong styles and I have followed several grand masters. I have become more confident in my practice. Yet all I can do is introduce you to the knowledge passed down from the experienced sages and what I have learned from my teachers. There are a total of 5,485 copies of Daoist books preserved, good condition or not, collected from all over China by the order of the emperor during the Song Dynasty (about 800 years ago). He ordered the best experts to update them. These books were preserved for research and practice to be carried out by posterity's scholars and practitioners. Until now, few scholar-masters have finished reading the entire body of work; very few works have been translated into foreign languages.

Chinese qigong is a profound and vast field that has developed into many schools; practitioners can start their practices in many different ways according to their condition. There are some types of qigong, both Daoist and Buddhist, that demand that the practitioners practice from childhood and begin as a virgin, such as Jin Zhong Zhao Gong, Qian Jin Zhui, and others; most do not have such demands. People who practice such qigong-martial arts will gain special powers regular qigong-martial arts practitioners cannot gain. Some martial arts masters decide to remain unmarried, or become monks or Daoists. Other types, however, allow the practitioners to get married afterwards.

## The Split into the Northern and Southern Daoist Schools

Sexuality and sexual intercourse are naturally included as important parts of qigong practice. Being a woman myself, I have always paid attention to information about female practice. Because there is no easy and simple way to define the role sexual activity plays in qigong practice, debates on the subject have been going on for more than a thousand years in China. There are different opinions on how to approach Dao. The debates between the different types of qigong experts has pushed sexual intercourse into a prominent place as an important health subject and has developed into a rich and broad scientific field in Chinese medicine.

The tradition since the very beginning of Daoist practice has included domestic Daoists who practice at home and do not necessarily belong to a monastery; their teachings has been passed in their families or disciples. The debates between two main groups of practicing became clearly evident more than a thousand years ago. The Daoists split into two major branches, the Quan Zhen School (or Qing Xiu, 1167 AD) also known as the Northern Daoist School and the "pair cultivation" known as the Southern Daoist School.

The main differences between the schools lie in their methods of cultivation in approaching Dao. Both groups have had their theories and practice forms handed down from ancient times. Both schools gradually developed more systematically during the Ming (1368–1644 AD) and the Qing (1644–1911 AD) dynasties. The debate between the two schools has involved many qigong practitioners in China up to this day. Both schools have produced many masters who have gained high powers and longevity, written excellent books, and produced immortals (celestials) during each dynasty.

The practice of the Southern Daoist School is for men and women to practice together, and is named "pair cultivation". In one of the Tibetan Buddhist Mi Zong Schools, the couple practice is similar to the Daoist pair cultivation practice. The first Dalai and Panchan's teacher, the great, erudite, and open-minded Mi Zong expert by the name of Tsongkhapa (circa 1300 AD) taught the practice. We may see the "splitting" as one way the sages opened more doors for the convenience of people and tailored the practices to the individual's aptitude.

### PAIR CULTIVATION IN THE SOUTHERN DAOIST SCHOOL

Since the Southern School practice is meant for couples, it is easy to confuse the pair-cultivation qigong practice with regular sexual intercourse or "bedroom skills." However, pair-cultivation qigong practice is for pursuing Dao, which is completely different in nature from using mere bedroom skills that yield good health, longevity, and a pleasant sexual relationship. With just good bedroom skills, you cannot attain immortality. The Daoist expert and scholar, Chen Ying-Ning told his students in the 1940s,

> The real Southern Daoist Pair Cultivation and the so-called sex qigong practice are as different as the clouds and the dirt. The understanding between the wrong and the right can be as tiny as only one-hair width yet the wrong understanding will lead the practitioner down the wrong path. One who teaches such qigong must have studied all nine types thoroughly before he can tell the true from the false. To practice this type, one must study all the nine types totally then he will be able to tell the true from the false. Otherwise, he will not just cause harm to self but harm others, too....You have to study and research and understand this profound theory first before you take action. You cannot just go ahead to try the methods without this foundation. Otherwise, it is like a scientist who repeatedly ignites the atom bomb without first understanding the theory, and doing the studies and research beforehand.

Chen warned that pair cultivation requires the right partner, location, money, and especially the right teacher. He also warned that to learn from someone who knows some of the theory but is not wholly qualified could be dangerous to health, even to life. He emphasized that since it is still taboo to talk about sex in the modern world, the teacher must be cautious when choosing a couple to teach. For a couple who is seeking the truth of life, sexual arousal is not simply for intimacy and pleasure, but is the best way to build up primary qi—it is a stepping stone to more advanced practice.

Because pair cultivation takes two persons of the opposite sex to practice together, there have been always bad apples who take advantage of such practice since ancient times. Not many real high-level masters of the Southern School have openly spoken out and corrected the wrong teachings, even today. I am sorry to say that the bad apples are mostly males, but there are a few female bad apples also. I call such people bad apples because they use qigong's name for sexual pleasure only or for money. A person who indulges in seeking only sexual pleasure will suffer consequences such as health problems. He will never experience the super pleasure described in my translation of a poem later in this chapter. There are also some deluded masters who believe that absorbing the essence from young female virgins can help them to complete their pursuit of longevity. Such masters, though few in number, can manipulate and lure naive females (and young men). It is impossible for these "masters" to pursue Dao because they act in opposition to Dao. These fake masters are held in contempt by the Chinese people. For these reasons, it is a good idea to educate yourself and learn only from a qualified teacher of good virtue if you do not want to be misled and want to practice advanced qigong.

From my consultation and discussion with two Daoist masters, the Vice Abbot of the White Cloud Monastery, Master and Dr. Li Yu-Lin (a man) and with the Abbess of Datong Xuan Zhen Guan (a woman who is the disciple of the twenty-ninth successor Dragon Gate of her monastery), I have found solid support for my research and my opinions expressed here. I am not going into great detail about pair cultivation because I do not have actual experience with it.

The term, pair cultivation (*shuang xiu*) was used by the Southern Daoist School when it was headed by Immortal Zhang Zi-Yang during the Song Dynasty (960–1279 AD). Immortal Zhang thought that to pursue Dao, a man and a woman—yang and yin—must practice together. Only when a man and woman cultivated together, enjoyed an appropriate sex life, and practiced correctly, could such practice prolong life. Together, the couple could form a complete path of cultivation to pursue Dao. Immortal Zhang's practice focuses mainly on the "gold dan." When referring to the practice, the Daoist term, yin and yang, is also defined differently by the two Daoist schools. To the Southern School, yin and yang means a man and a woman who practice together—the pair cultivation. If the couple succeeded in the practice, they were called an Immortal Couple, a term that is still used today by regular people to describe a beautiful and intelligent couple in an intimate relationship. There are, however, single practitioners in this school.

The theory in the Southern Daoist School is that to pursue Dao, one does not necessarily have to become a monk or a nun. Many ancient sages have set examples. Before the Jin (1115–1234) and Yuan Dynasties (1271–1368), according to the Daoist Master-scholar Hu Hai-Ya and the Buddhist Master-scholar, Nan Huai-Jin, ancient Daoism did not encourage a man to leave his wife and to avoid sex completely in order to achieve high-level qigong because it is against human nature. Master Nan thought that in light of what we have learned about internal secretion and hormone fields in modern medicine, this school can be considered very advanced scientifically.

Many well-known immortals were and are not religious Daoists, but people like you and me, and many high-level qigong masters of today have families and children. From several books that I have read, when pair-cultivation reaches a certain level, the couple can practice from a distance without touching each other and still can form a qi-energy field. My research tells me that pair cultivation is a period of practice. Eventually, the practitioners must practice alone.

## THE NORTHERN DAOIST SCHOOL

A brief translation of *quan zhen* is "tranquil and alone cultivation." Its meaning goes deeper than this as you will discover soon. The Northern Daoist School is considered to have originated from Zhuang Zi (the sage who came after Lao Zi). The school became the largest group during the Southern Song Dynasty in north China. The Northern School theory mingled Daoism with Buddhism. Northern School Daoists believe that yin and yang reside within one person. This is the principle of the practice handed by Immortal Wang Chong-Yang (1112–1170 AD) who established the Northern School. Practice in this school focuses on a return to human origins. Wang's principles are to live a simple life, practice thrift and simplicity, cease worrying, kindliness, submit to one's circumstances, make peace, be moral, and do good deeds. According to Immortal Wang Chong-Yang's definition in his poem, "Quan Zhen" means that the xin (heart-mind) has become clear about the truth of life and seeing nature. The poem reads,

> *The qi and blood circulate to transform without draining; the jing and shen mingle, but are no more fluid; the light of wisdom shine the three merged internal lights, the fortunate longevity has helped the person rise beyond the world.*

Another immortal during the Yuan Dynasty, by the name of Tushan Gong-Lu also defined Quan Zhen. *He wrote,

> *Quan means nothing is lacking or dirty, completely full; zhen means the infinite power that the person has explored but although he is capable to change whatever, it is not the truth; only Dao is real.*

Although the Quan Zhen School was named this way in order to show its different stance from the Southern Daoist School and its similarity to the theory of Buddhism, both schools have very different practice forms for approaching Dao. There are also some different opinions about how Immortal Wang attained high-level Dao. His students believed that the Immortal Wang's two teachers were Immortal Lu Dong-Bin and Immortal Zhong Li-Quan. Some experts thought Wang attained Dao in his own practice by his own wisdom and his diligent practice. Immortal Wang had seven disciples who all became important Daoist masters in history. People call them the Seven Quan Zhen Immortals. One of them was a female, Immortal Sun Bu-Er, who will be introduced in my next book on qigong for women.

One of the most influential Quan Zhen branches, the Dragon Gate Daoist School, was established by the youngest of the Seven Immortals named Qiu Chu-Ji. He developed the Quan Zhen theory and practice. His Dragon Gate Daoist School firmly promoted the theory that a person naturally had both yin and yang within, and there was no need for a different sex partner to participate when pursuing Dao. Both males and females have to go through the same

---

*Tushan was his family name. Most Chinese last names are one word with some exceptions.

period of harvesting the dan before reaching the level of immortality.

Although there are important differences between the Southern and Northern Daoist Schools, they both have a similar way of attaining Dao, that is, to cultivate and not attached to the material world. This is also the best set of principles in making progress in qigong practice. On the path of pursuing Dao, a practitioner needs adequate means of support to give him or herself the freedom to devote to practice, and to be aware of the necessity of not being attached to material things. In a poem written by the Sixth Buddhist Chan Successor, Master Hui-Neng says "All the happiness is in a one-inch square of field called xin (heart-mind). One can seek and to feel from there, there is will, there is communication."

After having briefly introduced the Northern and Southern Daoist Schools, I would like share with you a conjecture of mine. A 5,000-year-old clay jar unearthed in the Gan Su province in China shows a meditating figure with a man's head, but a woman's body. Does this drawing mean the yin and yang reside inside the same person? Perhaps this drawing of a male/female figure is trying to tell us that the result of high-level qigong practice is the interchangeability of the sex of male and female. In many Chinese classic novels, it is told that high-level masters were able to change their sexes. The celestials produced from both the Southern and Northern Daoist Schools—and the Buddhas from the Buddhist and Confucian types of practice—all can change into males or females. For example, Guan Yin, the Bodhisattva, is a male statue in the Tibetan monasteries; in mainland China, the statue is a beautiful female. According to the classic Buddhist books, Guan Yin was a male Buddha before our earth turned into the Ice Age. He appeared on the earth as a woman because "he" sympathized with the females who suffered more in many cultures in the world. I once read an article written by a well-known young master who was taught by such a male/female master in middle China.

## Practical Advice about Sexual Practices

HANDLING SENSATIONS

The Daoist expert Chen Ying-Zi, who passed away in 1996, instructed one of his students about entering the period of practice

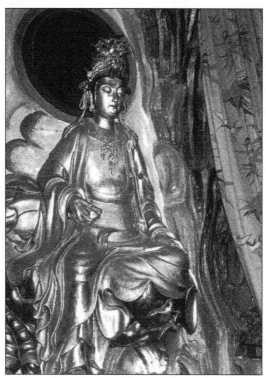

*Guan Yin's statue in Baima Monastery with a history of more than 1,900 years.*

(of sexual arousal during meditation described earlier) as well as the guidance about life. He emphasized that one should "not do [the practice] in a harsh way, but gradually." He gave an example, saying that

> ...if a rich man is also good at making money and managing, he can afford to waste some; if a rich man is not good at managing and wastes money, eventually the money will be gone. If a well-to-do man is good at making and managing money, he can become rich. If a poor man is in the same way, he can become well-to-do, maybe rich. But if a poor man is not good at making money, even if he does not waste, he is still poor; if he wastes, then we all know his end. This is called "broaden the source of income and reduce the expenses". [He thought it was important] to eat right to get plenty nutrition; breathe in the right way through the nose to absorb qi and to absorb qi  through the pores of the skin.

According to qigong theory, when a sensation that is similar to sexual arousal occurs in meditation, it indicates that plenty of qi that had accumulated inside is beginning to find a way out, that is, qi becomes active. At this point, the practitioner should shut the anus and private parts gently so that the qi does not leak out of the body. As a result, the qi rises up. If the practitioner handles the qi correctly, the sensation will promote the progress; if not, it can cause harm.

One goal of practice is to transform sexual arousal to essential energy. To do so, the practitioner should inhale very gently and almost imperceptibly give some attention to moving the qi energy to the area that is a bit beyond the lower dan tian, keeping it there for a short time until it is stable. Then in a very gentle way, the practitioner should bring the energy to the Wei Lu point (tail bone area) and move it up along the Du channel (along the spine) to the back of the head and send it into the Yu Zhen points (under the skull) to let the energy itself shower naturally through the brain. The way of sending the qi along should be done very gently. The sensation can be hot and there may be some noises in the head. The qi will then move from the top of the head down along the Ren channel (the middle of the chest), which is cooling down. When the energy passes the nose, the practitioner should gently hold the breath so that qi does not leak through nasal openings. All these movements need knowledge, experimentation, and long experience in qigong practice, especially meditation practice.

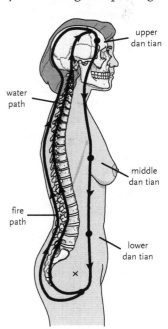

*Movement of active Qi.*

There are special qigong forms created by great masters for different purposes such as forms designed for repairing physical damage caused by intercourse, for treating sexual diseases, or for promoting affectionate sexual relationships, vitality and longevity. There are also practices for guiding strong and heated sexual desire into essential energy to build up health. The following quote taken from the book, *The Chinese Secretly Handed Down Precious Classic* written by a Daoist master of the Southern Daoist School who was one of Mao's private physicians, Zhu Heh-Ting gives advice on how to handle the sexual sensation when it occurs in meditation.

> *Dao between a couple originates from yin and yang; the origin of yin and yang is Dao. The fountain of Dao is qi. Qi and blood are from the organs... and the originator of the body is the shen of the xin (the spirit of the heart-mind). Love and passion from the xin create passionate communication and touching, which lead to a life-long closeness. So, passionate intercourse and affection is a natural tie between male and female.*

The Daoist belief is that only when both partners are pleased and satisfied, with the health of both be improved, will yin and yang be balanced and nourished. Otherwise, it will not be beneficial to either one's health, especially not to the only one who enjoys the act. Such practice is called bedroom skills, because it merely focuses on health and longevity. For a couple seeking a healthy life, sex is not simply a pleasure, but also a relationship. Bedroom skills can help a relationship. Sex is also inseparable from Traditional Chinese Medicine and diet.

According to Traditional Chinese Medicine and qigong theory, a happy mood produces *yang qi*—positive energy. The *Dao De Jing* written by Lao Zi says "a healthy, appropriate sex life could preserve and induce longevity and happiness, adjust and balance yin and yang, and preserve health." A documented record, Han Shu (chapter Yi Wen Zhi ) and a book unearthed in the 1970s from the Ma Wang Dui Tomb (both records were written during the Han Dynasty, 206 BC–220 AD, or earlier) contain details written about sex and longevity practices. One chapter was written in a question and answer form by Emperor Yao, the leader of the tribal society that existed before the time of the Yellow Emperor. Someone consulted Emperor-Sage Yao, "Why does the human's sex organ becomes old earlier than the rest of the body?" Yao answered that, "...the organ is used so frequently, but is not nourished and not used in the right way." Emperor Yao also explained why intercourse should be done in an appropriate way and the necessity for proper methods and skills. He responded to ten questions on how to cultivate longevity and enjoy good, healthy sexual relationships. He said, "When a couple is engaged in sexual intercourse and both are going to come, the man should inhale the woman's breath and keep his organ all the way down inside the woman without moving."

In modern Chinese laboratories, it has been proven that during this "going-to-come and inhale" moment, such practice can increase the concentration of carbon dioxide in the male's blood and help prolong his erection so as to please the female.

The Emperor then continued, "The man's organ should move in and out slowly, deeply, and slow down especially when pulling out, so that he can enjoy the pleasure and benefit both at the same time...because both are satisfied..." The Yellow Emperor, a sage-physician from about five thousand years ago, had a qigong teacher, Peng Zu, who also taught him qigong, sex, and longevity practice. Important medical books later written by the great Daoist physicians-and qigong masters such as Bao Puzi (Jin Dynasty, 284–363 AD), Dao Hong-Jing (Tang Dynasty, 456–536 AD), Sun Si-Miao (Tang Dynasty) all emphasized and explained the importance of a healthy and harmonious sexual relationship in ways that could prolong couple's lives. They all included specific sexual practices in their writings. These ancient sages built the foundation of longevity practice and of Traditional Chinese Medicine and diet. This is why longevity and the subject of sex are still considered to be closely related topics. These topics developed into a systematic, dialectical field in Chinese medicine, diet, and practice. Based on this theory, many tonic herbal formulas and diet recipes designed by well-known Daoist-physicians for building up the qi and jing energy to prolong lives were produced. All these originated from the same qi theory of Daoism.

Although most of the recipes and forms were written for men, both men and women can share many of them. Eating foods and taking herbal products are not as simple as it is shown in the media. Not knowing the nature of the foods and herbs and how they complement each other, or not using them correctly can cause harm. A tonic can be harmful if you take too much or use the wrong kind. These concerns are also expressed in the Chinese medicine and qigong books. In a word, such Traditional Chinese Medicine formulas and diet can play the role of "helpers" to build up both the man and woman's health while they enjoy a harmonious, pleasant sex relationship. This of course will benefit a qigong practitioner. Since my focus in this book is on qigong, and not Chinese medicine and diet, I have gathered some recipes for another book on herbal foods for longevity and vitality I hope to publish.

According to ancient Chinese qigong books, the time when couples make love can make a difference in its efficiency. The book unearthed in the Ma Wang Dui Tomb says that when a couple makes love at night, the man's *jing* [essence] would be more energetic and the love-making would benefit the female more; to make love in the morning, the result would be on the contrary, the female's jing would be more energetic and it would benefit the male more.

## Concerns About Qigong Practice and Sex

Generally speaking, all types of qigong can build up yang energy, but there are also many practices designed just for building up yang energy and for treating illnesses that cause impotence. Before we begin describing the practices, I express several concerns about what can go wrong in such practices.

A. A large concern of some Daoists with whom I talked is that some people confuse qigong practice with bedroom skills. Bedroom skills aim at health and longevity. In qigong practice, it refers to the sensation that occurs in the meditation state.

B. A serious concern is that some people either misunderstand qigong practice or there are bad apples who take advantage of women. The belief that gathering qi from young virgins could prolong lives is considered to reflect a lack of yin morality and can cause harm.

C. The concern of ignorance: According to health traditions in Daoism and in Traditional Chinese Medicine, although most of qigong practices do not demand abstention from intercourse; judicious moderation is beneficial.

D. The concern of unbalanced energy between the couple: If only one partner enjoys sexual intercourse, it is not healthy. Only when a couple has a mutually passionate sex life, will it benefit both partners' health. If only one of the two enjoys, eventually the sexual relationship will harm his yang energy after a long period of time. Those who do harmful things when seeking sexual satisfaction will eventually only harm their own health because such activity does not yield a balance between yin and yang.

E. Overdoing can harm health and shorten life. Those who seek endless sexual pleasure "will end up dead in a muddle-headed state" according to the immortals. The consequences of excessive intercourse are qi blockages and deficiency. The man will consume himself and harm the yin energy in his kidneys; as a result his yang energy will be affected. This situation causes disordered qi-blood circulation. Symptoms of the disorder are that he often feels dizzy, has tinnitus (ringing in the ear), feels weak in his waist and knees, feels tired, becomes forgetful, and exercises his judgment more slowly. His face color grows dim, and he may have sexual impotence. For a female, excessive sexual activity can bring about problems like disordered menses or leukorrhea, pain in her lower abdomen, prema-ture aging, or loosened teeth. All these occur because the kidneys are harmed, thereby lowering their immunity. In explaining the theory that excessiveness in sex will harm health, we can use the yin and yang picture and think of the white side as the living life period and the dark side as the death period. In the life side, the pleasure in one's sexuality is a part of nature. If the pleasure becomes too overwhelming and is overdone, life will automatically turn into the dark side—death. Because of this yin and yang theory, Chinese culture does not encourage masturbation because it is considered neither normal nor healthy. According to Traditional Chinese Medicine theory, frequent masturbation is harmful to health, especially to young boys because their bodies have not totally developed and physical development is adversely affected. Losing too much seminal fluid can cause the child to have sleep disorders, dizziness, memory impairment, listlessness, and even pathological changes in the other organs. This seems to be contrary to some American doctors' opinions. But also, several American researchers now share similar concerns. The American media reported in 1997 that several researchers thought that excessive intercourse could cause one's internal secretions to become disordered. They found that a harmonious, healthy sex life can help a couple live healthy and longer lives, which corresponds with ancient Daoist theory.

F. It is also considered not healthy if a man is constantly aroused and he must try to force himself to control his urges and not ejaculate. Several years ago, I read in a Chinese medical article about this. It said that in such a case, it could cause cancer in the man's prostate gland.

G. According to the ancient teachings by physicians in China such as Sun Si-Miao, it is considered unhealthy for a couple to share the same bed, but not make love over a long period of time. In such a case, the ancient physicians suggested that it would be better for them to live in different rooms. When a man tries hard often not to be aroused when lying next to a woman, his health will be harmed.

H. Men who have diseases should focus their qi to curing their illnesses and may need to avoid having sex for some time.

I. Warnings in classic Chinese medical books say that a couple should try to avoid making love when the seasons are changing, when there is a thunderstorm; when there is a lunar or sun eclipse; when one is exhausted, outraged or overjoyed, or when drunk.

J. There have been frauds perpetrated by qigong "masters" who are not at high levels, but pretend to have become an "immortal." A qigong practitioner should also know that not every religious Daoist or Buddhist monk is a well-educated high-level qigong master or a Traditional Chinese Medicine physician.

## Bedroom Skills for Prolonging Healthy Lives

The title of the chapter, "Sex and Longevity" in the book *The Chinese Secretly Handed Down Precious Classic* by Zhu Heh-Ting, clearly tells the reader that the chapter belongs to the realm of bedroom skills. I have translated some methods described in the book and from other sources in order to give you a hint of what the ancient sources say as well as help broaden your knowledge in achieving a healthy relationship and lasting lives.

Anyone can practice parts A and B. Do not just proceed with the practices in part C and beyond because health problems such as the tangling of the qi circulation may occur. If practitioners have qigong experience and do the parts from the earlier sections cautiously, and knows how to resolve a "tangled" qi problem, they can make the attempt to do parts C through E. Please remember to use these steps as references because such practice needs much education on qigong.

A. **Avoid draining too much energy.** To not drain too much energy when you are making love, hold your mind gently in your heart when the semen is ejaculated so that you are not overwhelmed and scatter your qi at the moment of coming.

B. **Warm up the kidneys.** Yang energy directly affects sexual ability. Before going to sleep at night, wear comfortable clothes, sit, and meditate for as long as you wish. While meditating, put your tongue tip up on the roof of the mouth at the maxilla, close to the teeth. After meditation, with your eyes closed, rub your palms together until they are warm and use them to cover the areas over the two kidneys. Then gently massage the areas at least 120 times.

C. **Emperor Yao's Methods.** This section was taken from *The Chinese Secretly Handed Down Precious Classic*. The man should hold his semen by deeply inhaling and exhaling three times, and at the same time contracting the anus five times in order not to come. He should then guide the semen gently to his brain along the governing channel (the Du channel along the spine) to the Yu Zhen points (under the bottom of the back skull). In this way, he would lose nothing, but gain more qi.

Chinese scientists have discovered that when a male holds in his semen correctly, the semen is absorbed in his seminal vesicle; his internal secretions are adjusted thereby making him energetic and stronger. This exercise needs to be taught by a good teacher because it is very important to do it in the right way.

From Xian Jing's article in Qigong & Science (6, 1996) we learn how both the man and woman can nourish each other during sex. When having intercourse, the male's organ should be deep down inside the female without moving. At the same time, he should imagine that there is an egg-sized crimson ball in the lower abdomen, while moving slowly in and out, but without coming. The female should visualize the ball as well. They should visualize that the ball stops moving right before the man comes. Before coming, this exercise should be repeated dozens of times. In the article, the author adds that this exercise helps stimulate the functioning of the sexual glandular system and promotes anti-aging. The man can also try sometimes not to come at all, so as to let the semen be absorbed as in the method described previously.

D. **From Another Ancient Book.** The man should exhale when going inside the female and inhale when pulling out. After repeating this exercise nine times, the man should then go all the way down as deeply as possible, and at the same time, his tongue tip touches the maxilla and his teeth are clenched. In this way, he will not become breathless. If he becomes breathless, he should stop and wait. Before coming, his mind should be at the lower dan tian (three fingers down the navel, inside close to the spine) and his organ should slowly play inside his partner. He should inhale and hold the semen, and at the same time, he should lift his anus and contract his lower abdomen while his mind guides the semen up into his brain along the governing channel (along the spine). At the same time, the female uses her mind to guide qi downward while the male guides it up along the spine, thus they form a circle.

E. **Lock the Gold Cabinet In the Dream Qigong.** This practice, which is for a hard penis that cannot return to its normal state, comes from an important ancient Daoist qigong form called Lock the Gold Cabinet In the Dream. This condition may occur in some male practitioners who have practiced for a long time and have accumulated plentiful qi inside. This method is for building up health and also for controlling nocturnal emission. It is not simply a method or a treatment; it is another way of creating a foundation for practicing more advanced qigong and is especially beneficial for young men. When using the practice to handle nocturnal emission, the practitioner absorbs his essence into the body. The practitioner should follow the steps gently and slowly with his mind.

Steps:

a. Gently keep the mind at the lower dan tian.

b. The mind is guided from the glans of the penis to the perineum, to the Wei Lu (tail bone), to the Jia Ji (approximately in the middle of the upper spine), to the Yu Zhen (under the skull), and passes to the brain to the front forehead area. Hold the thought at the upper dan tian (inside the front brain) for a while.

c. Your mind then guides the thought to the middle dan tian (inside between the nipples). While swallowing saliva at the same time, use the mind to guide the saliva going to the middle dan tian; while keeping the teeth clenched, the mouth closed, tongue tip touching the roof, your hands clenched into fists, and the toes of the feet are gripped tightly.

d. Repeat three times, and then return to the normal state.

# CHAPTER 8

# Qigong Exercises and Refining Qi

## Preparation

A human body is designed to mingle qi power with the power of nature and the universe. Qigong teaches us how to monitor the qi "engine." Whatever the qigong form—Daoist or Buddhist—they all process the refining of qi inside, thereby preventing illness. As a Chinese ancient teaching says, "Eating right to prevent diseases is better than to taking medicine to heal; practicing qigong to stay healthy is better than eating right to prevent illnesses."

Qi morality is used in qigong practice to soothe the emotional disturbances that can affect the practitioner's qi channels from circulating during practice. Although Daoists and Chinese Buddhist monks practice qigong, in many ways their practices in fact are related to the science of the human body and to cosmic science. Both share the same fundamental theory of human bodies and nature, such as the seasons and hours that can affect practice. Understanding this is the first step in beginning qigong practice. Although our environment has changed tremendously since ancient times, our inborn nature remains the same. No matter what type of qigong you practice, remember that qigong originated from ancient ways. The practice can help open up the qi channels, cleanse and heal, nourish the qi inside, and absorb more qi from nature.

### THE FIRST STEP

To a beginner, the first basic and important step is to maintain a relaxed, peaceful state of mind when you practice. Relax your whole body, especially the parts that are ordinarily tense. Relaxation allows your body to absorb qi from nature and gives the most freedom to your own "Doctor Qi" to heal you. If you cannot calm yourself down, go look at some beautiful scenery or talk to people so you can change your mood. Before starting to practice, keep one pleasant thought.

### REMEMBER THE IMPORTANCE OF PREVENTION

Whatever goal you have, cultivation is the kernel in qigong practice. Cultivating daily will help you become more relaxed; your mind becomes more at ease and is not as easily controlled by emotions. Daily practice cultivation can give you courage and guide you through life. We may call cultivation a tour guide that helps us to stay on the right track. The pleasant feeling of doing a good deed can promote qi circulation because "feeling nice about self" can increase positive energy—the yang energy inside.

A good experience for me is to write in a diary, not necessarily daily. I have found that a diary is like a mirror to remind me of some of my stubborn bad habits; I can check the wrongdoings and thoughts and record my progress. "To seek the reason" was a suggestion given by Immortal Lu to his students that I take seriously. Forgiveness and tolerance are the best ways to refine the qi inside. As a result, both the healing and practice progress more quickly. In someone with a large heart, qi has plenty space to travel and takes action with authority. The best way to exercise the heart is to work on solving the most sensitive and most difficult issues in life. To work on them but not avoiding them—as if purposely rubbing the sensitive spots with some salt—such as family problems that no one can avoid all. For example, learn to appreciate your own parents because they gave you a life and raised you. To respect parents was the advice given by all Chinese ancient sages, Lao Zi and the Buddha himself.

### LEARN THE GUIDANCE AND THEORY OF THE FORM

The best way to start your practice is to find a good teacher who is knowledgeable about qigong theory and forms. If there is no such teacher available nearby, and you must learn from a book or a tape, better get both. You can find reliable information from Internet web sites such as The Qigong Association of America (www.qi.org). Follow the guidance strictly in your practice and do not attempt to be creative. Any type of qigong can benefit health through self-effort. To feel when practicing is more important. Diligent practice is the key to healing.

### AVOID ILL THOUGHTS

A qigong practitioner must avoid any ill thoughts and negative emotions while practicing—qigong increases the movement of qi, but emotions disturb the qi movement. If, for example, you practice while you are in a bad mood, you create two "troops" fighting inside you that will only confuse your qi channels and send the negative energy that much more quickly to your organs. Any ill thought can cause the practitioner health problems because ill thoughts carry toxins that can harm the organs and qi movements. Ill thoughts can lead a qigong practitioner who has revealed extrasensory ability to the wrong path away from Dao or become deluded. The higher the power revealed, the more trouble and danger can occur if the master does not work on his own xin (heart-mind). Health problems, even delusions caused by ill thoughts, can be corrected by the practitioners themselves. The way is to retain one's own *shen*—the awareness and faith in a gentle way—and the need for correction will be recognized. This is why checking the inner thoughts daily can prevent such situations. Often, keeping the feeling of sunny-clear weather inside oneself helps. A positive attitude can also prevent unhealthy thoughts.

### READ AND STUDY, BUT DO NOT BELIEVE BLINDLY

Educating yourself and making informed decisions can avoid misunderstanding and prevent unhealthy thoughts. Read to educate yourself so that you will be able to tell which teachings are false. Nevertheless, you do not necessarily gain deeper understanding by studying or reading endlessly. Deeper understanding comes through your own experiences in persistent practice, as well as through awareness and mastery. Daoism defines qigong practice as a way "To master the opportunity and timing of your intermingling, the integration of qi, and cultivation of your qi; watching its changes gently and nourishing it; learning the skills of mastering the levels and degrees of qi to refine it." This definition can be understood only after you have experienced the qi movements as a result of long practice and studied qigong theory. Only then, if you are not satisfied merely good health, gaining some healing power, or revealing some low-leveled extrasensory ability, can you march on the journey of your life experiment.

## CHOOSE THE RIGHT TEACHER

To pursue high-level practice, one must have a qualified teacher and seek help. If you are seeking a grand master for advanced practice, you must learn how to choose a good teacher. Learn from different masters and also see their human sides. All the sages, including the Buddha himself, had many different teachers. The great Tibetan master, Ardixia, had 153 teachers and Tsongkhapa (1357–1419 AD) had more than 30. You must be cautious, however, if you want to become a disciple of a high-level master. Do not be a blind believer as in the Chinese parable of those who "lit incense and worshiped whichever temple they visited." Examine the teacher's morality, education, and the people who surround her. Good teachers follow the principles of Daoism or Buddhism; they do not violate the Buddha's or Lao Zi's teachings because no one else in our world has reached beyond the Buddha's and Lao Zi's level. This is why the right teacher will always carry out their masters' teachings exactly.

A high-level master will have an easy manner, a kindly face, a peaceful demeanor, an unselfish will, and will care about people. Some sources say about such a master that,

> The middle of his forehead looks full with a vague aura and
> has healthy skin. When this master is around, he makes
> people feel good. His fingernails can also tell you something
> about him or her. Their color is healthy, and if they look
> pale purple in color, they have gained the power to commu-
> nicate with immortals.

Rinpoche, the Tibetan Living Buddha Luosangtudanpai pointed out that the best teacher is from one's own *ding*—when all the wandering thoughts have been driven out and the practitioner retains a tranquil and calm manner, and wisdom begins to emerge.

## END THE PRACTICE CORRECTLY

To end a qigong moving form or to end a meditation in the right way is very important. Otherwise, you can drain your qi. It is like harvesting after you have grown your crops. Most of the forms have an ending method. A common and safe ending way is to mentally tell yourself that you are going to end the meditation. At this point, you may turn your tongue in circles to produce more saliva, and then divide the saliva into portions. Swallow slowly each portion into the lower dan tian and visualize the qi moving down together with the saliva. Use your mind to condense the qi there into a marble-sized qi ball in the lower dan tian. Someone may question whether the saliva can really go down there? The answer is, it does not matter. The more important purpose is to guide the qi down and condense it. The qi moves together with your body fluid. If you gather saliva and send it down to the lower dan tian often during the day, you will calm down. When you swallow the saliva, always slightly contract your bottom as if you were having a bowel movement. Do not contract hard because this could cause constipation later. Never focus too hard or too long on a particular area. When keeping the mind at an area, do so gently and very slightly. The chapter "Cautions" in my *Qi, The Treasure and Power of Your Body* gives advice on how to handle qi movements.

IF YOU FEEL DROWSY

Some people feel drowsy and even fall asleep when they meditate. This must be avoided. It is important to be vaguely awake and aware during meditation because when you feel the qi dropping, you must shut the perineum gently, and softly inhale to prevent the energy from being drained. At this point, you can relax. There are several ways to avoid drowsiness. You can choose one of them and try it for a short time. If it does not work, you may try another.

A. Stop the meditation and go to sleep or, better yet, make sure to have enough sleep before you meditate.

B. Open your eyes slightly and look at the end of your nose for a while. Avoid sitting there like a piece of wood thinking of nothing and your mind becoming numb, feeling nothing.

C. Master Nan Huai-Jin's teacher, Grand Master Yuan Huan-Xian taught people to visualize a small red light inside the navel, then shooting the light up to the top of the head, spreading its radiance.

D. Gather the strength of the whole body, and then shout "pei" loudly.

F. With the fingers, hold your nose until you cannot hold your breath anymore, and then breathe out hard.

G. Simply move your body or walk around until you are feeling totally awake and alive.

## Practicing the Forms

When practicing a form, moving or still, that has some mind work, the practitioner should try not to focus too hard. Mind (-heart) belongs to the Fire element according to the Five Element Theory. If mind work is overdone, it will be like overcooking a meal and burning it. My suggestion is to always practice some void-minded meditation (described in more detail later in the chapter) when practicing the meditation forms that have some mind work. The term "quiet and still form" is used only to compare with the forms that include movements. In any type of meditation, knowledge, posture, and relaxation are all important. If one of these is missing, a problem can arise. None of the above, however, will be important to a very high-level qigong master. I have chosen the following ancient forms from the best practices that have been used for thousands of years up to today. According to my experience, they are safe and proven to work effectively. You may choose one from the following methods to try.

### For exercising qi

Inhale slowly, evenly and softly through your nose all the way down into the lower dan tian until the lower abdomen is full. Hold your breath gently and count from one to 90 at the rhythm of one count per second. If you cannot hold on for this long, let out a little breath but try not to let out much, and then keep holding your breath and your body relaxed. Or do the breathing gradually to add repetitions. After counting to 90, maybe even more if you can, exhale through your mouth as slowly and softly as you can while your mind mentally sends the qi up to your hair and down to your feet. When doing this, hold your thoughts so the qi does not scatter.

This method strengthens your bones and tendons. Also, after you practice this form persistently for a long period of time, you will not feel hungry.

### The Six Exhaling Sounds Exercise—To cleanse the organs

The ancient Daoist Six Exhaling Sounds Exercise is a good method for cleansing, building up health, and opening up the channels. There are also different ways to coordinate the exhaling sounds practice with some simple movements. In general, do each from six to thirty-six times, depending on your health. After practicing for a long time, you should feel the qi flowing to different organs when you inhale. The sounds are:

*Heh–* (heart-Fire) *Hoo–* (spleen/stomach-Earth) *Sss–* (lung-Gold/metal) *Chwee–* (kidney-Water) *Xu–* (liver-Wood) *Xi–* (gallbladder and the San Jiao—Three Warmers).

When starting this practice, you should inhale and exhale as quietly, long, and thoroughly as you can; make each sound six times. Always tighten the perineum (hui yin) slightly when you exhale to make the sounds and also when sending qi into the lower dan tian while inhaling. At the same time, place your hands on the sides of your legs and gently form empty fists. You can do this in a sitting posture, lying down, or standing. When standing, your empty fists lay naturally on the sides of your legs. When lying, put your fists slightly away from the sides of your legs, near the middle line of the pants, facing downward. Or, you can put your middle fingers so they touch the legs gently. When sitting, lay the empty fists on your knees. You may make one sound more times if you have a weak organ. Follow the arrows in the Five Element chart. For instance, if your lung is weak, do more *Sss–* sounds. You can also nourish the Earth element in order to help the Gold/metal. Exhaling to make a sound helps to release the toxin in that organ and inhaling helps absorb qi to build up the organ. For this reason, the deeper the inhalation, the more qi that is absorbed the better. Some practice the whole form facing one direction to the sun in the early morning,

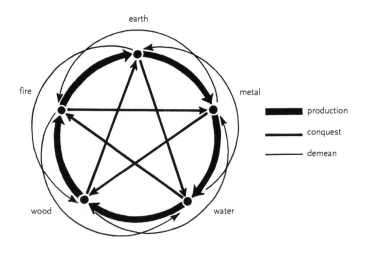

*The Five Elements.*

others practice and move facing the different directions according to the Five Element Theory, all depending on one's need and comfort level. When you choose one way, stick to this way and experience the practice fully.

Steps

a. In the morning while facing the east, stand with the feet set to the width of your shoulder and relax the whole body.

b. Inhale through the nose slowly, softly, and continuously. While inhaling, gently use your mind to send qi all way down to the lower dan tian, at the same time gently contracting the perineum (hui yin).

c. When the qi you inhaled all goes down to the lower dan tian and you have gently contracted your anus, start making the Heh– sound through the mouth softly, slowly, evenly, and thoroughly until you have totally exhaled, but are not breathless.

d. When breathing out totally and finishing the sound, repeat, if you can, the first step. If you cannot, relax your whole body and then begin the first step again

e. Begin to inhale as described earlier, and then exhale to make the same sound so softly that you yourself cannot even hear it. Repeat this six times or more. Generally, do no more than a total of 36 repetitions. If you have certain severe diseases that you think will benefit from doing this practice, you may exhale the sounds for more than 36 times. But never exhale more than 120 times; otherwise you will drain your qi.

### For longevity

Do this exercise whenever you can. Visualize the reddish-purple rays of the sun coming to your mouth and nose and inhale the rays slowly until your mouth is full of light. Then swallow saliva all way down to the lower dan tian 27 times and contract the perineum (hui yin) very gently while swallowing. Repeat this four times. This exercise prevents illness and improves your skin tone.

### For longevity and preventing evil

Frequently visualize that there is an egg-sized, golden shiny qi ball in your heart area. It should be golden on the outside and red inside. You can also simply visualize that your heart is like a bright and shiny fireball.

## THE BODHISATTVA (GUAN YIN) DA MING INCANTATION (SIX INCANTATIONS)

Tibetan people chant these six sounds daily. The incantations originated with Guan Yin—Avalokitesvara, the beautiful woman's figure of a Bodhisattva. (In Tibetan paintings, she appears in a male form.) The pronunciation of the six incantations are:

*Wung–   (m)Ar–   Mai   Bei–   Mei–   Heng–*

I have compared these pronunciations in several books written by high-level Chinese masters, including a Tibetan and a Mongolian master. They all sound the same, except the *Mei–*. Some masters write it as Nei. In this book, I use Mei, the way that I learned from Grand Master Wang Zi-Shen, a disciple of a well-known Tibetan Master Monk. From my own research, either one will work well if you persist with the chanting.

Before chanting, take a deep breath through the nose slowly, softly, all way deep down to the lower dan tian first. The soft way is as though you are smelling a flower and nobody can hear you inhaling, including yourself.

The best way is to chant all six incantations without stopping in the middle during chanting. When finishing the sixth sound, continue with exhaling, inhaling, and chanting.

Start from the first sound, one by one, each lasting as long as you can make it. At the same time, imagine you are like a full moon, crystal clear, and clean inside and out.

When chanting the last sound, *Heng–*, think of the sound as rising up to the throat, and then up to the head in the third-eye area (inside the head, about half of your index finger deep). Or just chant and focus your mind gently on the sounds.

Chant seven times at least, the more the better. Chant out loudly or quietly depending on the situation. As for your posture, you may either have your palms closed into a prayer posture. If you are in the sitting meditation posture, place the palms together with the thumbs touching. Just let the mind focus on chanting. Chanting helps open up the middle channels, clear all the qi channels, and promotes the circulation of qi and blood for healing and preventing illness. The chanting can also prevent evil spirits, especially when you chant in a stern tone. My other qigong books include additional material about the Six Incantation practice.

## To "EAT" QI

**Form A.** This is a partial pi gu practice.

a. In the morning or before 1:00 P.M., stand near a pine, cypress, or fir tree, and relax for a while.

b. Inhale slowly, softly, and evenly through your nose. At the same time, imagine all the pores of your body opening up, and then hold your breath gently while visualizing that yang qi (or good qi) is streaming in through the pores.

c. Hold your breath as long as you can. When you cannot hold your breath anymore, visualize all the pores slowly closing and all the qi that you have absorbed moving into the lower dan tian where you condense it into a marble-sized ball.

d. After the qi ball is made, begin to exhale slowly, gently through your mouth with your perineum slightly held.

Repeat from a to d as many times as you wish.

**Form B.** In the evening, imagine that you are swallowing the stars and the moon into your lower dan tian. The method can be compared with a turtle stretching its neck to open its mouth as if gargling food from the air.

## Meditation

### TIMING YOUR MEDITATION

Meditate whenever you can because it will always benefit your health. Timing can mean "all the time"; "the right time" inside the body; the time to coordinate with nature, that is, with the environment and the stars. Choosing the right hour to meditate can increase its benefits for most qigong practitioners. For many people, the time during the day when you always feel most energetic will be the right time. According to Traditional Chinese Medicine and qigong theory, the blood and qi channels in our body become more active during different hours (noted here as military time). For example, between 23:00 P.M.–24:00 midnight, the qi and blood in the gallbladder channel is more active and plentiful, making it a good time for people who have gallbladder illnesses to meditate. Between 1:00 A.M. and 3:00 A.M. is good for people who have liver problems; between

3:00 A.M.–5:00 A.M. for lung illness; 5:00A.M.–7:00 A.M. for large intestine problems; 7:00 A.M.–9:00 A.M. for stomach illnesses; 9:00 A.M.–11:00 A.M. for the spleen; 11:00–A.M. to 12:00 noon for the heart; 13:00 P.M.–3:00 P.M. for the small intestine; 3:00 P.M.–5:00 P.M. for the gallbladder; 5:00 P.M.–7:00 P.M. for the kidneys; 719:00 P.M.–9:00 P.M. for pericardial disease; 9:00 P.M.–11:00 P.M. for san-jiao problems (*san jiao* means the heat in the head or stomach).

WAYS TO ENTER THE MEDITATIVE STATE

You may choose from the following list and consider your own condition and personality. The immortals taught their disciples different methods of meditation according to how they thought the individuals could best benefit. The following are chosen from different sources and are just suggestions.

A. If you are a type who thinks too much and it is hard for you to focus, use the counting method. Count from 1 to 10, then repeat, focus on counting until you are totally absorbed in the meditation and can forget counting.

B. For illnesses related to the liver, such as gallbladder, eyes, and tendons, focus your mind on the Da Dun point (0.1 cm from the right bottom-corner of the big toe nail of your right foot).

C. For illnesses related to the heart, such as small intestine, blood vessels, and tongue, focus your mind on the Zhong Chong point (top of the middle finger).

D. For illnesses related to the stomach-spleen, such as digestion, blood deficiency, diarrhea, constipation, and blood illness, focus your mind on the Zu San Li (three fingers below the kneecap outside part).

E. For illnesses related to the lung channel, such as the large intestine, skin, and nasal passages, focus your mind on the Shao Shang point (0.1 cm away from the outside corner of the thumb nail).

F. For illnesses related to the kidneys, such as gallbladder, urinary tract, bones, and hearing, focus your mind on the Yong Quan point (bottom of your feet, upper middle).

G. For those with low blood pressure, brains deprived of blood due to yang deficiency, and fear of cold, focus your mind on the Bai Hui point (top of your head). To find the Bai Hui

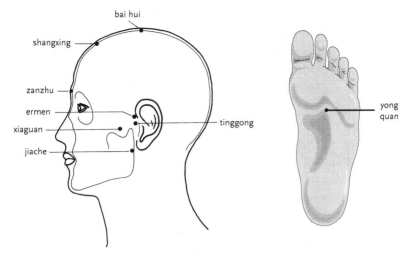

*Some useful Qigong points.*

point, use your thumbs to touch the top of your ears and touch your middle fingers above your scalp.

H. For normalizing the heart-brain function and preventing problems related to the nervous system, focus your mind on the Lao Gong point. To find the point, bend your middle finger to touch the palm.

I. For promoting the circulation of qi and blood, which is especially helpful for females, focus your mind on the Shan Zhong point (between the two nipples).

J. For uneasy people who feel that it is difficult to focus the mind inside one's body, they can focus on something outside, such as red flowers, green trees, green mountains, or white clouds. The subject should be pleasant, soothing, and not overly stimulating.

FOR THE BEGINNING MEDITATOR

Beginning level meditation can be relaxing. You must avoid becoming chilled or wearing overly warm clothes when meditating. You must not let anyone or anything startle you. You can do your meditation standing, lying, or sitting positions and different styles that match certain types of practices. The meditative state looks quiet on the surface, but the qi motion can be very active inside the body. Meditation is a very important part of any type of qigong practice. It is, in fact, the foundation as well as the ladder for more experienced qigong practitioners who pursue advanced stages, and is the sole way to pursue Dao. To practice long hours of advanced meditation, the practitioner must be experienced, knowledgeable, and understanding. If you want to pursue advanced practice, you must learn meditation from a qualified teacher. This teacher should not just have a certificate, but should be someone that you know for sure can instruct you well.

The popularly used practice of simply "emptying your mind" technique is in fact not that simple. A practitioner must have a good understanding of the "simplicity;" it takes much work to arrive at that point. The sages created many ways of meditating. Their purpose was to let the mind focus on one thing, and the ultimate purpose of all meditation is to refine qi within and reach the void state. This multifold approach was taken because humans are complex beings with different personalities and who have minds that are very difficult to empty. Simplicity is in fact not that simple.

Different types of qigong may share similar methods in their meditations and also may have unique features. For example, the fixed *mudra* (the hand's postures) can differ. The hand's postures, which are like antennas used by different radio stations, help you tune into the energy of the celestials, immortals, and the universe more quickly. The most common meditation posture is to sit with the legs folded with the palms together at the lower dan tian area touching the thumbs gently. Usually the male's left hand lays on top of his right palm while the female lays her right hand on top of her left palm. In this way, the qi flow forms a circle around and inside the body. Choose one practice for a period of time, stick to it, and take the time to feel it fully.

FOR THE EXPERIENCED MEDITATOR

For most practitioners, meditation is the sole way of becoming enlightened—to attain Dao at the beginning level. When a qigong practitioner has no more thoughts floating in and out, no longer feels the physical body's existence, and yet does not feel drowsy, she has successfully entered a deep meditation state. This state is the void state, in which the practitioner is always in control always during deep meditation. If the practitioner continues to practice like this, someday, internal breathing can happen spontaneously. In this type of breathing, the practitioner naturally stops breathing through the nose; instead she breathes through the skin.

This state is called "the unity of the universe and human being." This state only happens after the practitioner has accumulated plentiful qi inside. In this state, it is very important that the practitioner is aware of the self still being fully in control. The state of mind is somewhat like half-sleeping. This practitioner experiences some physical sensations and perhaps some phenomena. This is the important time when the practitioner should keep in mind that whatever happens, not to fall into blind worship or be fearful. The sensations or phenomena come from her mind. Now self-cultivation is at work. Self-cultivation prevents the practitioner from being led astray by her own ill thoughts. Study and cultivation helps the practitioner who seeks spiritual growth. These preparations are not only for attaining a profound understanding of simplicity and reaching the void state, but also helps to prepare the practitioner have a good understanding of any possible extrasensory activity that may occur during meditation. Only when this person maintains such understanding, the time of learning the truth of life comes. Eventually, the practitioner reaches the point where there is no more need of books and she can be instructed by a teacher and guided individually. Such a teacher can come from anywhere, even the most unlikely people. Again, choose one practice for a period of time, stick with it, and take the time to feel it fully.

MEDITATION FORMS

**For general health:**

A. You may put a statue or a painting of Guan Yin or a Buddha in front of you, gaze at the image for a while, and then close your eyes. Visualize that he/she is meditating in the same posture as you, and contemplate the aura surrounding him/her for a while, then move him/her into yourself and become him or her while you meditate. You can meditate as long as you wish. Do not forget the ending method when you decide to end the meditation.
Remember, avoid worshipping anything you "see" in the Buddha in front of you. You are just borrowing an image to help you enter the meditative state when you start. You are still your own master.

B. You can chant to help yourself enter the meditation state. Chants were passed on from the ancient sages who gained Dao. Chanting helps you forget the real world. Also, the ancient chanting sounds function like the antenna of a radio station that help to tune up the qi energy. Chanting can help you to receive more energy from the universe and tune up inside. The different sounds can affect different parts of the body when you chant them. You can use the Six Incantations described earlier in this chapter.

C. You may gently observe your xin—visualize your heart-mind—and hold this thought very gently, even when walking around all day long. You can also focus your awareness in the heart area or in the middle point between the two nipples deep inside close to the spine, or even focus on the point under the ribs inside the hollow point, under the sternum. Ignore any qi activity because when you use your mind, the qi will follow your mind. As a result, the qi doctor's work will be interrupted.

D. You may listen to the sounds of water: water fountains, rain, streams, rivers, ocean waves, or breezes, or listen to your own heartbeats, but with an absent yet gently attentive mind.

E. You can have thoughts while meditating, but the way differs from daily thinking. You should gently let your thoughts in and cultivate and figure out what is the right thing to do and what was done wrong. Then let the thought go like a piece of white cloud, not at all attached. Maintain that void space in a gentle way, until the second thought floats in. Then think in a gentle way and retain in the state either as before or simply let it go, again keeping the space void until the third thought floats in, and so on. Generally, to meditate for twenty minutes to two hours is enough when practicing for health purposes. Do not force your mind to empty.

F. After sunset, lie on your back, relax, and imagine that there is a sun on your forehead and a full-moon under the navel.

**For preventing senile dementia:**

A. The senior can visualize that there is a small ball like a setting sun at lower dan tian; it moves in slow motion turning in forward-back-forward circles.

B. The method of visualizing lights inside originated from a well-known doctor, Chao Yuan-Fang in the Sui Dynasty (581–618 AD). During the Tang Dynasty (618–907 AD), Princess Wen Cheng who was married to the Tibetan king brought his book to Tibet. The following is a partial practice for seniors:

Visualize a reddish light at the heart area for about 15 minutes. Then, gradually for about three minutes, imagine spreading the light to the entire body. If you do not have high blood pressure, gather the light to the top of the head for about two minutes.

To end the practice, gather in all the light very slowly and gently down to the lower dan tian, and meditate in the void state of mind for about two minutes. All the timing and periods can be flexible.

For seniors who have high blood pressure, they can simply gather all the light to the lower dan tian, which is about three fingers down the navel, deep inside the lower abdomen close to the spine.

# CHAPTER 9

# The Healing Power of Qigong and Modern Chinese Medicine

Qigong heals because it teaches its practitioners how to coexist harmoniously with others and how to follow the the laws of nature to survive and adapt to circumstances. For example, during some unusual seasons, older or weaker people often die because their bodies have become weak and have lost the ability to adapt to the changing environment. In contrast, senior qigong practitioners rarely die during the same seasons because qigong practice helped their bodies adapt to natural changing conditions.

According to qigong and Traditional Chinese Medicine (TCM) theory, in the spring, the liver is stronger and the spleen weak; in the summer, the heart is stronger and the lung is weak; in the autumn, the lung is stronger but the liver is weak; in the winter, the kidneys are stronger but the heart is weak.

The kidneys are considered to be the essential root of life, and yet they are more easily harmed than the other organs in all four seasons. The vulnerability of the kidneys and their loss of balance leads to many, if not most, illnesses. The word "kidney" in Chinese medicine does not simply mean the organ, but also the growth and development of the brain. The kidneys act as the major organ for regulating water metabolism, controlling discharge of urine and stool; it also cooperates with the lung and spleen. The kidneys control the private parts including the lower dan tian area (inside the abdomen, three fingers down the navel). The kidney essence, the term used in qigong and Traditional Chinese Medicine, which is considered to develop life, originates from the conjugation of the

| | WOOD 木 | FIRE 火 | EARTH 土 | METAL 金 | WATER 水 |
|---|---|---|---|---|---|
| DIRECTION | East | South | Center | West | North |
| SEASON | Spring | Summer | Long Summer | Autumn | Winter |
| CLIMACTIC CONDITION | Wind | Summer Heat | Dampness | Dryness | Cold |
| PROCESS | Birth | Growth | Transformation | Harvest | Storage |
| COLOR | Green | Red | Yellow | White | Black |
| TASTE | Sour | Bitter | Sweet | Pungent | Salty |
| SMELL | Goatish | Burning | Fragrant | Rank | Rotten |
| YIN ORGAN | Liver | Heart | Spleen | Lungs | Kidneys |
| YANG ORGAN | Gall Bladder | Small Intestine | Stomach | Large Intestine | Bladder |
| OPENING | Eyes | Tongue | Mouth | Nose | Ears |
| TISSUE | Sinews | Blood Vessels | Flesh | Skin/Hair | Bones |
| EMOTION | Anger | Happiness | Pensiveness | Sadness | Fear |
| HUMAN SOUND | Shout | Laughter | Song | Weeping | Groan |

*The Five Element Theory.*

innate reproductive essence of both sexes and the foundation of reproduction. The kidneys are related to aging and affect the bone, bone marrow, and hearing.

Qigong practice can restore balance in the body. Qigong theory teaches people how to eat correctly, how to sleep well, how to rest, how to work, and so forth when adapting to the changing seasons. Qigong is not merely a set of deep breathing exercises or even a method of controlling breathing; it is a profound human science that gives you freedom from having to seek health care. Qigong, in fact, is the science of natural health care. What is more, qigong is the only "doctor" working for no recompense, for adapting to the very different needs of its practitioners, and the only method that meets the needs all types of health issues.

Qigong is also important because qi and qigong contains a human sensibility that can help people with their emotions and to get in touch with their souls, something medicine or technology often lacks. According to a story in the Chinese newspaper, *Beijing Daily*, some stolen items were even returned to their original owners after the thieves learned qigong. People involved in qigong not only become healthier, but also become wiser and nicer. And qigong practice can lead to a huge reduction in the amount of money spent on health care.

## Qigong Practice and Modern Experiments

Now that we've explored many aspects of qigong, let us take a look at how modern Chinese medicine takes advantage of ancient wisdom and practical experience gained over thousands of years to arrive at innovative ways to use qigong in their modern medical practice. Qigong often helps physicians go beyond what is offered by conventional medical practice.

Qigong's use in healing and medicine has gained recognition in the United States only recently. In 1997, the vice president of a large New York publishing house rejected this book saying that he had never heard of qigong. Between the lines, I sensed the word, "quackery." Later that year, *Newsweek* published its first article about qigong. More and more Americans began to hear about qigong over the next few years. Most beginning practitioners of qigong in the West know little about how qigong actually works. Others are waiting for scientific proof that qigong works. For these reasons, I will describe some of the work on qi and qigong being done by Chinese researchers. When describing the experiments, I have included the places and institutes where the experiments were performed, and listed other relevant citations and information whenever possible. Most of the experiments and clinical treatments were originally described in Dr. Feng Li-Da's books and in the *Qigong & Science* magazine. In the reference section, I added other sources, mostly in Chinese, that describe the experiments and clinical treatments in more detail. What I present here is only a partial sampling of the rich literature that is available in Chinese.

We often hear that someone died of a heart failure or kidney failure. In other words, when one important organ dies or fails to work well, this person usually does not live long. Qigong practice can repair an organ and its parts by normalizing and readjusting the entire body. When you practice qigong consistently, a gradual readjustment of your biological clock occurs. In this process of reversing biological clock, your skin will automatically look younger and smoother; this is one example of how qigong practice slows down the aging process. That qigong practice can slow aging has been documented in many ancient Daoist books and classic novels.

Qigong exercise strengthens the joints, tendons, and muscles and promotes the blood-qi circulation. Spiritually, qigong practice soothes the heart-mind (xin) and helps practitioners become more peaceful, calm, and centered. In this way, the qi inside builds up resulting in the enhancement of the practitioner's immune system. Qigong is a method of prevention as well. I am an example of this. For over ten years, when I begin to feel that I am catching a cold, I have always stopped the cold by using the qi inside me, eating right, and occasionally using an herbal formula. That a cold has seldom taken root in me is one of the benefits of my longtime qigong practice. Preventing illnesses is one of qigong's most important functions from which millions of Chinese qigong practitioners have benefited. Prevention of illnesses, anti-aging, and qigong practice all work to prolong a healthy life. According to qigong theory, a human's life span can be prolonged; the actual length of life depends on whether the person has accumulated large quantities of qi. When a person's qi is plentiful, she will be strong and live a long life; if there is little qi build-up, the person does not enjoy good health and her life span is usually shorter. Qigong is the best way to cleanse, adjust, and build up qi inside the body, not just absorbing qi through practice. More importantly, qigong is the sole way to accumulate and store qi.

Experiments in China have shown that qigong can improve the pineal gland's functioning and increase its melatonin hormone secretion. This increased melatonin might be one of the reasons that qigong can prolong life. Researchers have discovered measurable temperature changes on a qigong master's skin during a meditation state. Also, qigong can slow the aging of the pineal gland and reverse our body clock.

In the following paragraphs, I briefly describe some medical and scientific research on how qigong acts, prolongs life, and improves the quality of life in seniors. Again in order to avoid confusion, I would like to emphasize that these descriptions of experiments are meant only to offer a glimpse into what is being investigated in China today. There is a large body of literature and research reports that is available only in Chinese. As much as possible, I've identified the hospitals and institutes where the research was conducted. Many of these reports were taken from the *Qigong & Science* magazine. If you wish to learn more, you can contact these places in China.

In 1992, scientists and researchers from the Canton Qigong

Academic Institute in China placed several plants, mice, and microbes in the same hall where grand master qigong practitioners were giving lectures and treating patients. The researchers found that the qi energy given off by the masters benefited humans, plants, and beneficial microbes, but killed the microbes that were harmful to plants as well as the mice. Earlier in the book, we learned that qi energy is indeed different from other types of energies because it has thoughts and "knows" where to go.

Other researchers used modern instruments to examine the places where high-level qigong masters lectured and taught qigong. Inside those places, strong qi-energy fields that contained a large quantity of elements were found. Professor Lu Zi-Yin of the Beijing National Science Institute used instruments to test the auditorium when there were several thousand people who were listening to grand qigong masters' lectures and receiving qi treatments at the same time. He found some motion of high-energy matter that resembled gamma rays; there were also detectable elements in the air similar to neutrons. These elements may have affected the audience and lead to some changes in their bodies. The researchers could not yet put a name to the nature of this energy and could only say that they were similar to gamma rays. These experiments are yet another example of what Westerners find difficult to readily accept at this time.

Another experiment was performed in 1992 on a very cold winter day (about 10 degrees Fahrenheit below zero) in Xiang Hong Qi, Inner Mongolia. After the researchers were assured by the grand qigong master, Dr. Yan Xin, that no participant would become sick from the workshop, they began their experiment: The audience was not told that the heat in the hall would remain off. Dr. Yan Xin lectured for twelve hours until four o'clock in the morning. Two weeks after the workshop, the researchers surveyed all participants and were amazed to find that none of them had caught a cold. In fact, they all felt more energetic. Several who had colds before they came to the workshop were even healed.

The phenomenal healing power of qigong has begun to convince people in the West. In March 1995, a Swedish physician took fourteen patients with severe hearing problems to Beijing to receive qigong treatments and learn qigong. After eleven days, the symptoms in eight patients were greatly reduced. In the same year, several American educators went to visit a qigong program for learning-impaired children.

Each summer, more than eighty students from Russia, Ukraine, Germany and Spain go to the Shaolin Temple with Master Xu Ming-Tang to practice qigong healing. In 2001, the number of students grew to more than 200. A few of Master Xu's students have even revealed scanning abilities; they can see through the skin and muscles, even down into the bones, something Westerners find difficult to believe.

Researchers at the Chinese Traditional Medicine Hospital in Gan Su province discovered that qigong practice can reduce oxygen consumption by 16%. As a result, the reduced oxygen consumption slows down the brain waves, promotes the activity of brain cells, increases the functioning of the nervous system, and improves the internal secretory system. The reduced consumption of energy increases the life of cells. Researchers found that qigong helps to reduce stress, an important factor in prolonging life. Their findings support the ancient theory that qigong practice produces and improves the quality of saliva. Saliva quality, in turn, has an important effect on aging. An extract from the saliva can be used to treat and reduce the symptoms of senile dementia. This finding supports ancient qigong practices that taught people to swallow saliva in a special way in order to increase the fluid in the gallbladder, pancreas, intestines, and stomach, as well as a means of aiding digestion. According to their research, qigong practice increases the practitioner's ability to absorb the most nutrition from food and gain greater amounts of calories from food than do people who do not practice qigong.

Researchers at the Hospital of Wu Han City in the Hunan province followed the effect of qigong practice on some seniors (*Qigong & Science 4*, 1995). The seniors who practiced qigong included cardio-cerebral and angiocardiopathy patients; those who had cervical spondylopathy, and those who had neurosis were compared with seniors who did not practice qigong. The average age of the seniors in these two groups was 58 years. The group who practiced qigong reduced their symptoms of sympatheticotonia markedly and improved their microcirculation. They slept better and their general health improved. Those who practiced qigong for a long time did not age as much as the non-practitioner group.

Doctors and researchers at a Beijing hospital followed two groups of practicing and non-practicing seniors in the Xuan Wu district and found obvious health differences. The senior qigong practitioners did not age as quickly as those who did not practice qigong. The qigong practitioners had improved blood pressure, more often had normal vision and hearing, as well as good memories. In contrast, the same measurements for the group that did not practice qigong were worse, fewer had normal hearing and vision, and a third of them could not do physical work.

Dr. Tang Mei-Tsi and her colleagues compared two groups of seniors in Beijing. One group of 122 seniors practiced qigong and the second group of 90 seniors who did not. The ages and educational level of the two groups were similar. Analysis showed that the senior qigong practitioners had much lower scores for the SDS (Self-Evaluated Depression) and SAS (Self-Evaluated Anxiety) tests than those of the non-qigong practitioner seniors. The qigong group also slept much better than the other group. Their movements were more stable.

Dr. Hu Song-Chang's research group reported that after three years of following two groups of seniors, he found that the group who practiced qigong had improved lung vital capacity, visual sense, gripping power, jumping, and feeling sense, and other abilities than the group who did not practice qigong.

## Qigong—Healing Illnesses

In China, qigong plays an important role in healing all kinds of conditions. Several qigong hospitals have been established in recent years for treating the mentally ill. An increasing number of qigong healing departments have been established in Western medicine hospitals. In another area of healing, qigong is used to help patients with physical disabilities accomplish self-adjustment with mind work by doing both moving and meditation forms. People with lost limbs or paralysis benefited from good qigong teachers who guided them. The rest of this chapter describes how such healing is accomplished.

**Eye Problems in School Children:** In all Chinese schools, qigong has been practiced in some form or other from kindergarten to high school since 1949, although most of the time nobody called it qigong. I did all those so-called physical exercises during my elementary to college years; only later did I realize that the movements were taken from qigong theory. The eye exercises used the acupressure elements and movements in which the acupoints and qi channels related to vision were massaged. In the physical education class, the teacher always told us to "breathe all way down to the lower dan tian."

Several Chinese journalists investigated how qigong was used to treat students with nearsightedness at the Railroad Elementary School in Xin Yang City, Henan province. The students were asked to do eye-qigong for three to five minutes daily over a period of four years. Before doing qigong exercises, among the 129 students, only 49 students had normal vision. At the end of four years, 96 students' vision became normal; eight students of the 25 students whose vision had been poor became normal.

The Tai Yuan City Qigong Treatment Center in the Shanxi province chose groups from two high schools and one elementary school to do an experiment on nearsightedness on a total of 176 students. All four groups did qigong exercises twice a day, one between the four classes in the morning and one after the classes were over in the afternoon. The students did the exercise by following their teachers, qigong audio tapes, or the doctor in their schools. Each exercise period was twelve minutes long. Each month, the students received eye exams, including the students in comparison groups who not practicing qigong.

After three months, the vision of over 40% of the students who exercised qigong was improved. In none of the students did their vision become. At the same time, these students improved their overall health, as well as their grades. For example, one ten-year-old boy, before doing qigong exercises, could not focus in class, often caused trouble, and disturbed the whole class. After four months of qigong exercise, he became a different person. He studied hard, made good grades, and got a B+ in both math and Chinese. Another ten-year-old boy had been timid and was often sick before he learned qigong. After four months qigong exercise, his mother reported that his poor digestion was much improved, and he seldom became sick. When experts met to discuss the results, they discovered that the younger the students were, the better the results. And better results occurred when the students followed the instructions carefully and were also relaxed.

**Learning-Impaired Children:** The teachers of Yun Nan University in Yun Nan province carried out experiments on 14 learning-impaired children who were 7–11 years old. The intelligence test (IQ) scores of eight of the 14 children were 35–49, and the rest were between 50–70. Their teachers taught them qigong forms designed for them four times a day, half an hour each time after the classes. The practice included both a moving form and meditation, plus some qi treatment. After two-and-a-half months, nine students had improved intellectually and five underwent no change. There was a nine-year-old student whose IQ (*zhi shang*) was measured at 46 before the start of the qigong exercise regime. Before she learned qigong, she could not copy Chinese characters, and her fingers were clumsy. After learning qigong, her memory improved, and now she is able to listen to the teacher in class and tell her parents about her homework. A ten-year-old boy who had an IQ of 70 before he came to this school is now able to pay attention and listen to the teacher in class. His memory also improved.

## TREATING MAMMARY GLAND HYPERPLASIA

In 1992, Dr. Yang Bian and Dr. Liu Zun-Xiang of Shen Yang Military General Hospital used qigong treatment to treat fifty patients who had mammary gland hyperplasia. The patients' ages ranged between 22 and 42. They had been ill for two months to five years. Their symptoms were mainly swollen and painful breasts that had one or more flat lumps. None of them had ever received qi treatments before, but had received other kinds of medical treatments such as herbs, drugs, instruments, acupuncture, magnetism or electricity. All had been ineffective. All the patients' symptoms were reduced or disappeared after three to six months of treatments. Their swellings and pain were gone. Among the 31 patient had had the growth in one breast, 23 recovered their health completely. Among the 19 patients who had the growths in both breasts, 9 recovered after they received qi treatments plus medical and acupuncture treatments.

TREATING CANCER WITH QI

The following descriptions describe how qiqong is used in China to treat cancer in ways that differ radically from Western approaches. According to Chinese medicine, most types of cancers are caused by emotions that have been repressed for a long time; this situation is thought to have caused stagnation in the flow of qi and the blood. Qigong used to treat cancer soothes the patient's emotions and relieves the stagnation. With such treatment, surgery is usually not needed and qigong is combined with diet and herbal medicine. That qigong has saved many cancer patients' lives is considered to be a fact in China.

Whenever possible, I've given some of the sources that describe these clinical experiments to enable the Western reader find the original citations and learn more about the qigong-based medical approaches used effectively in China. Before you read about the cases, remember that according to qigong theory, a life has a natural ability to absorb energy and this is why a human body can undergo self-repair. When qi is supplied by a qigong master, the cells absorb this healing energy.

A. **Carcinoma of the Uterus/Metrocarcinoma:** Dr. Feng Li-Da and Dr. Ju-Qing Qian divided samples of cancer cells into two parts. One part received qi treatment from a qigong master for 20 minutes, and the other part did not. The treatment destroyed an average of 31% of the cancer cells. The experiments were repeated 20 times, and in 18 times, the rate of the cancer cells destroyed ranged between 15–36%.

B. **Adenocarcinoma of the Stomach:** After a one-hour qi treatment on another set of cell samples with this type of cancer, one quarter of the cancer cells were destroyed. The hairs on the surface of the cancer cell visibly shrunk or disappeared; some cells had holes, and others died. Dr. Feng and her colleagues also observed changes in the chromosomes of the adenocarcinoma cancer cells. They repeated the qi treatments ten times under the same conditions. They found very different changes between the two groups of cells, in which one group received qi and the other group did not.

C. **Cancer in the Abdomen:** A suspension of cancer cells was collected from a case of a patient with cancer in the abdomen. In three trials, a qigong master gave a qi treatment to the suspension. The growth rate of the cancer cells was reduced by approximately 35% in all three trials.

D. **Cancer Prevention and Treating Malignant Tumor Cells:** Dr. Feng Li-Da and her colleagues divided 29 mice into three groups: one group did not receive qi treatments, but received cancer cell transplants; the second and third groups both received qi treatments for two weeks before the transplant. Afterwards, only the third group received qi treatment for two weeks again after the transplant. Two weeks after the transplants, the researchers dissected the tumors in the mice and weighed them. The reduction of growth rate in the cancer cells for the three groups were: first group, none (used as the baseline), second group, approximately 20%, and the third group, 32%.

These experiments show that qi treatment can control cancer cell growth at least temporarily. Dr. Feng said the experiments did not actually prove that short-term qi treatment can normalize the entire body, including body weight, and improve the spleen, but did show that short-term qi treatment can control cancer cell growth. Dr. Feng is planning experiments to show that long-term qigong exercise can make all organs change. "Note that this does not mean that qigong cannot induce immunity," she emphasized in her book, *Modern Qigongology*, "A large number of experiments have shown that qigong practice induces immunity and normalizes the whole body, and there are no side effects as with medicines which are used for improving only one organ and which then disturbs the balance of the whole system."

E. **Cervical Carcinoma, Stomach Cancer, and Ascites Carcinoma:** Dr. Feng and her colleagues repeatedly observed qigong masters who gave qi treatment to cancer cells. All cancer cells in these experiments were then compared with cancer cells that were not treated by qi. The following are three results:

Twenty repetitions of several qigong masters giving qi treatments on cells of cervical carcinoma: Approximately 31% cervical carcinoma cells died or were destroyed, and in

18 out of the 20 repetitions, the rate of cancer cell death ranged between 15–36%.

Forty-one repetitions of one-hour qi treatments by several qigong masters on cells of stomach cancer: Approximately 25% of the stomach cancer cells were destroyed and killed after the series of one-hour treatments.

A qigong master repeated the ten-minute qi treatments on the ascites carcinoma. The rate of control of the growth of cancer cell growth was approximately 35% in all three experiments. Qigong masters gave qi to a mixture of body fluid of which the density of cancer cells was 340,000/ml.

**Terminally Ill Cancer Patients:** The originator of Tai Chi Wu Xing Gong, Grand Master Heh Bin-Hui was invited in 1994 by the National Qigong Research Institute to treat cancer patients at a 21-day workshop in Beijing. All the patients were terminally ill and many were already at a critical stage. The terminally ill patients diagnosed by their doctors were told that their lives could not be saved. More than 78% of them were cancer patients. Master Heh studied the patients' records, talked with many of the patients and some of their family members, and then designed his treatment plan. First, Master Heh and his five students organized a powerful qi-energy field before giving the qi treatment. He requested that the patients go on pi gu—not eating food, but learning to absorb qi. The patients were told to learn and practice qigong for at least six to seven hours each day.

Before the 21-day workshop began, the cancer patients were examined thoroughly and after the qigong treatment, they were examined again by the same doctors. All patients were thoroughly examined, except for two cases. One of the two was a patient whose breast cancer had metastasized to osteocarcinoma (bone cancer) and the other was a lung cancer patient whose cancer had metastasized in the brain. The doctors were surprised to find that almost all the cancerous tumors shrunk significantly. In the next paragraph, two interesting cases are described in more detail.

Patient One had a malignant tumor that shrank from 2.8 x 2.4 cm to 2.2 x 1.8 cm in her abdomen. Patient Two, a 76-year-old male came to the workshop one week late. After the workshop, the carcinoma of a rectal polyp and two kidney stones all disappeared. Before treatment, his urine had contained a reddish sediment. After the workshop, his urination became normal as it had been five years before. Five days after the workshop, some dark hair grew on his bald head, many of his senile plaque disappeared, and his facial skin became moist and shiny.

After the workshop, the doctors and qigong masters who designed continuing treatments decided to use a Daoist qigong, with the goal of preserving health. The qigong healer blocked several acupoints of the patients by using a qigong method to "surround and annihilate" the area, and then gave qi treatments. Fifteen days comprised one treatment period. The qigong masters requested their patients to follow these steps:

1. They guided the patients during a sitting meditation, relaxed with their eyes closed for 20–30 minutes.

2. They asked the patients to move both their hands to the lower stomach, and wait until their palms began to feel warm. Next, the patients were instructed to imagine sending the heat into the stomach for a while. The patients were told to move both their hands in a clockwise circle 26 times; and then move their hands 36 times in the counterclockwise direction. Finally, they were told to push the hands out and pull them in several times.

3. The qigong masters asked the patients to move both hands up to the Shan Zhong point (middle point between the nipples), and then separate the two hands and cover the two nipples without touching them. With fingers slightly apart and bent, both hands were told to move in inward circles for three to five minutes; and then both were told to move in outward circles for another three to five minutes. Next the patients were told told to form both hands into fists, and move them clockwise 36 times, and then counterclockwise 36 times.

4. They asked the patients to move their hands to the kidney areas, push and pull without touching their bodies; and then move the hands to the front along the upper ribs, above their heads with palms facing upward, back to the kidney areas, and then pull and push again. They were told to repeat this portion many times.

5. Afterwards, they asked their patients to sit and meditate in a bathtub full of water for ten to twenty minutes.

During the treatment period, qigong masters also gave qigong treatments to adjust the patients' bodies. These treatments were given in various ways and were based on the patients' conditions.

In 39 patients out of 50, the flat lumps disappeared, and there was no more pain. In seven patients, the patients made great improvements, experiencing either no more pain or reduction in the size of the hyperplasias. In 4 cases, the patients had their pain reduced, and their hyperplasia's sizes were reduced to less than half. No patient experienced lack of improvement in one form or another.

TREATING HARDENED AND INFECTED TENDONS AND MUSCLES

Dr. Ding Hou-Di of Shanghai (*Qigong & Science 10*, 1994) used qi to treat acupoints to adjust the hardened and infected tendons, and muscles of patients. He treated three male patients who were in their thirties. The patients had reached advanced stages; their bones were achy, their movements were affected, and they all had been treated in the large hospitals without being helped. As their last hope, they went to Dr. Ding's clinic. Masters who had solid qigong training gave the following treatments.

1. The patient was asked to lie on his stomach with both arms in front of his head, to relax, to meditate, and to cooperate with the qigong doctor. Doctor Ding stood on the left side of the patient and used Yi Zhi Chan Gong to press both Fen Chi, Jian Jing, Tian Zong, Qu Chi, Wai Guan, and He Gu points on both sides of the body. Next, he used his thumbs to give a qi massage along these points from the patient's head to neck, to shoulders, arms and to the He Gu points. At the same time, he did tui na and qi massage. He repeated all these treatment three times on each patient.

2. Dr. Ding's two thumbs pressed the Bladder Jing channel along the spine from top to bottom, seven times. Then he asked the patient to exhale when pressing down and think at the same time, "Qi moves around my whole body, all parts and my four limbs have become relaxed and soft." Next, Ding asked the patient to inhale slowly when relaxed.

3. Dr. Ding used Yi Zhi Chan Gong again to press the Dei Bian, Huan Tiao, Ju Niu, Wei Zhong, Chen Shan, Kun Lun and Tai Xi points on both sides along the hip and legs of the patient, and then he used both thumbs to do tui na and qi

massage along the Huan Tiao and Ju Niu points to the back part of the thighs, and along the sciatic nerve down to the tendons of the heels. Next, he lifted and pinched the acu-point areas with his fingers. He repeated the whole treatment three times on each patient.

4. Dr. Ding asked the patient to lie on his back. He formed his fingers to look like claws before doing a qi massage and tui na along the chest bones from top to the bottom on both sides. He did this seven times on each patient.

5. Dr. Ding used Yi Zhi Chan Qigong to press the Pi Guan, Xue Hai, Yang Ling points, then he bent the patient's knees and waist areas and asked the patient to think at the same time, "My legs and waist are relaxed and loosened up. They are healthy and move in a nimble way." Dr. Ding repeated this treatment seven times.

All three patients had satisfactory results. For example, one patient who had been ill for three years had been forced to retire early. His previous hospital examination report showed the curvature in his spine and his chest was obviously not straight. His pain was significantly reduced after the first treatment. The patient then began learning a type of qigong in Dr. Ding's hospital and received treatments at the same time. After 37 treatments over a two month period, his symptoms had tremendously improved. His whole body's stiffness softened, as did his spine and his joints. He was able to bend down or kneel down, and go up and down stairs. Now he is able to take care of himself and return to work. Half a year later, the results were still stable.

CHRONIC BLOOD PRESSURE PROBLEMS

Dr. Wu Long-Chang of the Canton Mao Ming Chinese Medicine Hospital used qigong to treat chronic blood pressure problems in 39 clinical patients whose ages ranged from 20 to 70. The longest disease history was 50 years, and the shortest was three years. Some of the patients had experienced pathological organ changes. None of them had received much relief from either drugs or herbs, and most of them did not have faith in qigong treatment. The blood pressure of all patients was lower than 86/56mmHg; one of the patient's was only 50/20mmHg. Dr. Wu treated each of them individually according to the theory of Traditional Chinese Medicine. Treatment was determined, for example, by whether the patient had spleen deficiency, or kidney yang deficiency, or qi and blood deficiency.

Over a twelve-day period, there was one treatment per day that lasted 30 minutes. Dr. Wu taught his patients to do meditation. Those who had blood deficiency were told to lie on their stomachs; the others were on their backs. There was no mind work, but they were treated with qi machines. Dr. Wu then himself used qi to check the patients, and gave them individualized qi treatment. He also worked on the patient's Ming Men points, lower dan tian, Zu San Li, and assisted working on the Da Dun to unblock Nei Guan, Fei Yu, Xue Hai points in addition to the San Yin Jiao, Yun Quan, and other points.

The blood pressure in 23 patients returned to normal before finishing the first complete treatment set. After the first treatment set was completed, blood pressure became normal in ten patients. After two complete treatments, the blood pressure in three more patients became normal. Another three patients recovered after three treatments.

## LIVER AND STONES IN GALLBLADDERS

Dr. Wang Chang-Yin (M.D.) of Jiang Su province (*Qigong & Science* 5, 1994) described his practice of using qigong to treat liver and gallbladder stones. He concluded that modern medicine could be helpless regarding chronic diseases, a conclusion based on his many years of conventional medical practice. He started treating gallstone diseases in 1986, and found qigong very helpful. His first patient, who happened to be very sensitive to qigong, was a 44-year-old countrywoman. After he gave her qigong treatment, she passed the stone the next day and totally recovered after ten days. During the qigong treatments, no other kind of treatment was involved.

Dr. Wu was encouraged by his first success and started experimenting more on his patients. He found that he could use qigong to treat patients who were sensitive or insensitive to qi treatment with good results. After a whole year's experimentation, Dr. Wu was able to help patients pass their stones within three days. In the following years, he has created a complete qigong form used to release stones successfully. He has trained many students who have cured more than 10,000 patients with a success rate of more than 98%. He was asked to treat 12 medical doctors in the Su Zhou Hospital who had lithiasis. Most of them had been his professors when he was in medical school. After Dr. Wu's treatments, eleven of them passed their stones in their stool. The twelfth patient forgot to check his defecate in the following days; his result could be not counted.

## Treating a Mysterious Disease

Sometimes a person will have an illness that cannot be easily diagnosed or treated. A twenty-eight-year old farmer from Chong Qing area in the Sichuan province suddenly became weak after catching a cold and overworking himself in the field. He could only walk short distances and his hands could only reach his mouth. He was taken to a hospital immediately. After receiving intravenous glucose drips and medicine, he became worse. Despite the laboratory tests, the doctors could not find the cause of his disease. His family took him to two more large hospitals whose doctors could not help him. It was evident that he was dying and his doctor agreed with his family to invite a qigong doctor, Liu Zhu-Qiang, to the hospital.

The patient felt better after Dr. Liu gave him the first treatment, and he stopped taking medicine. After the second and third treatment, his condition was much improved. After ten days of Dr. Liu's qi treatment, the patient could walk up and down stairs by himself and take care of himself. He returned home and received qigong treatments five times at home. After a total 15 days of treatments, he recovered almost completely and started working in the fields again. Now he has learned to do qigong himself.

## Treating Injuries in Athletes

Dr. Yu Zhu-Tian, an experienced sports doctor, has been using qi to treat injuries. His work on 100 cases (70 male and 30 female players, aged between 12 and 17) is described here. The young athletes were divided as follows: 25 track and field players, 20 ball players, 12 gymnasts, 7 martial artists, 2 wrestlers, 10 racing boat players, 8 fencers, 7 judoists, and 9 boxers. The qigong doctor gave qi treatments through the needle at the A Shi point; he treated the injured muscle area, the depth and breadth of the affected muscles, and the strike joint for 20 minutes.

The results differed because of the different types of qigong that the qigong doctor practiced or the amount of qi power that the qigong doctor was able to deliver. Each athlete received one to three treatments according to the case. The more relaxed the patient, the better were the results. The table below indicates that the treatments usually resulted in complete healing and substantial improvements in the body part that was injured.

| Body Part Affected | Healed | Much Improved | Improved | No improvement |
|---|---|---|---|---|
| Arm | 12 | 12 | | |
| Leg | 26 | 20 | 2 | 3 |
| Shoulder | 14 | 14 | | |
| Waist | 28 | 18 | 7 | 3 |
| Other | 20 | 20 | 20 | |

It is interesting to note that the Chinese government has also employed qigong masters to train and treat athletes, including soldiers and police officers. One marathon runner said he felt less tired and ran faster after he used qigong methods in his running. Sports medicine in China is well-established field that makes good use of qigong healing.

SHOULDER PROBLEMS IN SENIORS

Dr. Li Si-Chen from Su Zhou City wrote an article in *Qigong & Science* (2, 1994) and summarized his many years of experience of using qigong to treat seniors' shoulder problems. He treated his patients individually and used different acupoints. All patients were healed or benefited greatly. The table (following page) shows the symptom, the acupoints treated, the length of qi treatment on each point, and the number of repetitions.

TREATING CORONARY HEART AND HIGH CARDIAC OUTPUT DISEASES

The Gan Su Province Qigong Research and Treatment Center used qigong to treat 139 cases of coronary heart (91 in one group) and high cardiac output (41 in another group) diseases; six patients had severe heart failure. The Center taught those patients two types of qigong, The Quick Way to Heal and Nine Steps to Keep in Good Health. There were 74 males and 65 females, whose ages ranged between 7 and 78. The longest history of illness in a patient was 22 years, from the age of 41, and the shortest history was a year and a half. The center has achieved comparatively better results than regular hospitals. The treatment plan was (described below) was carefully designed to make the best use of qigong methods.

| Symptom | Acupoints treated | Minutes each acupoint received qi treatment | Number of treatments given |
|---|---|---|---|
| Shoulder pain | Jian Yu, Jian Zhen, Jia Zhong Yu, Xiao Hai | 5 | 1–3 |
| Shoulder joint pain | Jian Yu, Jian Zhen, Yun Men, Yang Ling Quan | 5 | 1–3 |
| Shoulder joint obstruction | Tian Zong, Jian Yu, Jian Zhen | 5 | 1–3 |
| Pain around shoulder joint | Ju Niu | 10–20 | 1–3 |
| Scapulohumeralperi arthritis | Yun Men, Jian Niu, Yang Ling Quan | 5 | 1–3 |
| Shoulder unable to do lifting | Wen Liu, Jian Qian, Qing Leng Yun | 5 | 1–3 |
| Shoulder heavy unable to do lifting | Jian Niu, Yun Men, Zhong Fu,Yang Xi, Tian Niu | 5 | 1–3 |
| Shoulder heavy with pain | Treat same points as the previous, plus Jian Jing | 5 | 1–3 |
| Shoulder injury and hand pain | Shou Zong, Jian Zhen, Que Pen, Er Jian, San Jian, Yang Ling Quan, Xia Lian, Jin Hui | 5 | 1–7 |
| Shoulder and arm pain | Da Zhui, Jian Yu, Lao Zhen, Qing Leng Yun, Xiao Hai, Guan Chong, Zhi Gou | 5 | 1–3 |
| Shoulder and arm involvement, unable to do lifting | Jian Ru, Qing Ling, Qu Jin | 5 | 1–3 |
| Shoulder, arm myotenositis | Bin Feng, Qu Huan | 5 | 1–3 |
| Shoulder and elbow pain | Pian Li, Wen Liu, Xia Lian, Shou Wu Li, Zhou Niu | 5 | 1–3 |
| Shoulder pain causing neck pain | Que Pen | 10–15 | 1–3 |
| Gouty shoulder | Jian Yu, Jian Ru, Jian Zhen, Tian Zong, Qu Chi, Shou Wu Li, He Gu | 5 | 1–5 |

1. Each month, the patients were taught to do the designated qigong treatments, and then the patients exercised together for 25 days. Each week, the doctors and qigong masters met to discuss the patients' conditions and decide whether the patient should continue to use the medicine or to reduce the doses, or to stop using medicine, and also if the type of qigong needed to change.

2. After ten days of practicing this type of qigong, the qigong master selected a specific healing-heart form (chosen on the basis of the patient's condition) and taught it to the patient in order to strengthen his self-healing process.

3. The qigong master organized patients who formed a qi-energy field for healing together.

4. The qigong masters treated each patient's different channels according to their specific cases for ten minutes. They also treated these spots, as well as the Bai Hui, Nei Guan, Shen Yu, Ge Yu points, and assisted with qigong massage.

5. After the qigong workshop, the patients went home and practiced qigong by themselves. Each month, the patients underwent medical examinations and the doctors checked their exercises. After 180 days, the patients were examined at the county hospital.

At the end of the treatment period, most of the patients' symptoms such as headaches, dizziness, hearing loss, palpitation, shortness of breath or chest pain disappeared or improved. They slept well, ate well, and their blood pressure, arrhythmia, blood lipids, EKG all became normal. The patients themselves felt well. Only one patient from each group failed to improve. The average triglyceride levels, the blood cholesterol levels, and pulse rate all decreased significantly.

## Medical Investigations on Qigong Treatments

The medical data that I have translated from the Chinese literature and reports may be of interest to professionals, as well as others who would like to know more about the benefits of qigong treatments. The descriptions presented in the next few paragraphs are simply translations from the magazines on qigong (for example, *Qigong & Science*) or from the internationally well-known Dr. Feng Li-

Da's book *Qigong in Modern Science.* I have not elaborated on the figures, preferring to simply present the information.

## Effect of Qigong Practice on Blood and Surface Temperatures

The doctors of the Chinese Space Medicine Research Institute, Hou Shu-Li, Wang Lian-Ron, and three other doctors tested 31 people who practiced different types of qigong for 1.5 to 2.8 years. Their ages ranged between 12 and 46. The qigong practitioners were asked to stay in the room that remained at a steady temperature and to lie on their backs. The doctors measured the blood oxygenation, blood pressure, and skin temperature before the practice session after being quiet for 15 minutes and when the patients had reached the qigong state. The findings showed that during the qigong state, the measures improved greatly. For example, the level of oxygen in the blood rose to as much as three times higher in the qigong state than its level before beginning the exercise.

## Changing the Blood and Capillary Circulation

Many laboratory results have shown that qigong can also change the blood's circulation (*Qigong & Science 3*, 1995). For example, qigong can adjust the blood flow from the heart to make the heart transfer the exact volume of blood that it needs. When a qigong master sleeps, the blood transfer automatically slows down and reduces the blood amount sent to the heart; this phenomenon does not occur in a person who does not practice qigong. Laboratory measurements showed that qigong could induce changes in the actual blood vessels, and make them much more sensitive and elastic. Many experiments have also shown that when people practice qigong, their capillary circulation in the whole body is improved greatly and their skin also becomes smoother and younger looking.

The Zhe Jiang Hospital in the Zhe Jiang province has repeatedly observed many patients treated by qigong masters. They found the number of blood cells of all patients increased after receiving qi treatments. The numbers continually rose afterwards because the blood-producing function of their body had been improved. The number of the blood platelets also increased. In contrast, when the healers were giving treatment to their patients, the healers' blood cells apparently decreased while they gave treatments. The healers can, however, raise their own level of blood cells after they practice qigong.

The hospital's laboratory experiments also showed that qigong can reduce high blood pressure. Qigong also can change the alcohol levels in the blood and thereby fight aging, and treat diseases that are related to blood problems, blood vessels, or tumors.

The hospital in Zhe Jiang and many other hospitals have found that sugar levels were reduced in the blood and urine of their diabetic patients who learned and practiced qigong. Many of their diabetic patients have recovered and no longer needed to receive insulin treatments.

The doctors in the hospital in Zhe Jiang found that patients who practice qigong or receive qi treatments can improve the trace elements in their blood serum. Among the fourteen kinds, the zinc level improves and rises greatly. Zinc affects the body and metabolism. Qigong theory indicates that zinc can increase the level of many trace elements in the body and that practicing qigong can prolong life.

QIGONG STATES AND BRAIN ACTIVITY

The following results come from Chinese hospitals and their extensive medical experiments on qigong practitioners and people who received qi treatments from qigong masters (*Qigong & Science 2*, 1994). These experiments show that when a person is in a qigong state, his brain cortex remains at a high-level state that occurs in a non-qigong person only for about a 14 to 16 second period during dreams. This is the period that a person's brain is in the highly self-protective inhibition state according to scientists. A qigong practitioner can extend this 14–16 second period to a longer time while in a qigong state. As a result, the brain cortex will get the best and highest quality rest period as well as a readjustment in the body. In qigong states, Chinese scientists discovered that the cells in the deeper parts of the brain of a qigong practitioner show an excellent excitation state, and then show a strong brain biological current. The strong biological current occurs in the spot that the person keeps his mind on. In this state, the mind guides the biological current to function more powerfully on the spot where the person's mind is focused on. This is perhaps why someone can suddenly recover some long-lost memory at that moment.

The experiments showed that when a person is in a qigong state, the colloid in the protein in her body fluid forms something like a microcosm, and then forms a charged microcosm, after which it is then mixed with the body fluids and gives off a current. As a result, the activity of the brain cells is strengthened.

Modern science has demonstrated that most of the human's brain cells are not used—even only 20% of Einstein's brain was used. Scientists estimate that there are 140–150 hundred million cells in a human's brain, and only 3%–10% are used. What is actually the potential power in the brain that we have not yet explored? The Chinese qigong sages and masters all were quite sure that human beings did have potentials in the brain that could be developed and explored by practicing qigong. If a person practices qigong, the cells in a person's deeper brain can be stimulated and made active, thereby increasing the brain's potential, energy, and functions. Many parts of a human being's body have potential functions that we now use, especially the brain cells.

Since qigong can strengthen the current of the brain cell, the functions of the right side and the rest of the brain, which contains the most energy, may be enhanced. That is how many qigong practitioners in China (as well as some of Dr. Yan Xin's American students in the U.S.) have gained certain extrasensory powers by practicing qigong.

Also, there are differences between men and women's brains. Not long ago, several American scientists and researchers announced their new discovery: men and women used their brains in different ways. They found that men tend to use the left brain more and women tend to use the right brain more. This discovery supports the 5,000-year-old qigong theory that there are differences between the male brain and the female's brain. The focus of the minds between men and women often can be different in qigong practice. The Chinese doctors diagnose men and women and emphasize their differences, such as showing more concern about women's emotions. I describe some of this in my *A Women's Qigong Guide.* Chinese scientists have also demonstrated that qi works on the genetic code, on minds, and on memories in the subconscious. By far the best definition about qi is found in ancient Chinese books such as the *I Ching* and *Nei Jing.*

Experiments have also indicated that when a qigong practitioner is in a qigong state, his EEG resembled the EEGs from youth or young children. Also, the capillary blood circulation in the brain was significantly improved. At the same time, his brain received a plentiful supply of blood, especially in the forehead area, which is considered to be where the "sixth sense" resides. This section of the brain enables the qigong practitioner to scan through another's body, or "see" through a subject, maybe a soul. This forehead area can acquire functions similar to instruments that scan our bodies. Not enough scientists take these extrasensory abilities seriously enough. We know that this forehead area does play a major function according to ancient qigong theory as well as the experiences of qigong masters who have revealed the functions of their third eye. This area is like a reflector, which can give off light and reflect the subjects it "sees." I have personally met such people and tested them.

Experiments also show that when a person is in a qigong state, his sympathetic nervous system continuously reduces its activity and readjusts; the practitioner's cranial nerves, including the nerve center, all undergo ideal adjustment and improvement. In this way, the readjustment helps patients who have sleep disorders, neurosis, or neurasthenia; they improve quickly after qigong practice. For those people who generally sleep well may sleep fewer hours but still feel as well.

Dr. Feng, Li-Da's colleagues from the Shen Yang Military General Hospital, including Dr. Zhang Jian-Zhou, looked at the electroencephalograms (EEG) of ten high-level qigong masters who had practiced qigong for more than ten years. The masters were tested before and after they practiced qigong. After eight minutes of practicing qigong, their EEGs were compared; the changes were obvious. Most of the changes occurred in the front part of their brains. The frontal section of the brain is considered by doctors and by qigong theory to have the most potential and the highest activity level. It is also where the "third eye" resides. At the same time, the researchers tested another ten healthy people who were not qigong practitioners. These people were asked to sit quietly and relax for five minutes, then imitate qigong movements for ten minutes, and finally sit and relax for five minutes. During the different periods, their EEG did not undergo noticeable changes, unlike the qigong masters' EEG that looked quite different. The experiment showed that the qigong masters' EEG in a qigong state occurred in regular patterns, but with activity taking place mainly in the forehead and front part of the brains. Such activity was different from what occurred in the state between sleeping and awakening. This state was not the inhibitory (nerve) state, but a special qigong active state.

In 1978, a researcher, Mr. Gu Han-Sen of Shanghai Atomic Nuclear Research Institute, tested qigong masters' brain waves. He and his colleagues saw a picture of taiji (the drawing of yin and yang). The picture was not as clearly outlined as in the diagram, but nevertheless is a taiji picture. Gu also tested another well-known qigong master, Lin Hou-Sheng. He used an instrument to measure Lin's qi from his palm and recorded the data. Then he recorded the qi energy that Lin emitted when he treated the Yang Guan point (waist area) on a paralyzed patient for 30 seconds. Gu compared Lin's power and the power emitted by a physiotherapy machine. The power from Lin was much lower than the machine, but the treatment results were more effective than the treatment with the machine.

Reading about the scientific and clinical investigations in China may help you understand why the Chinese have never forsaken the old healing methods during the so-called "high civilization" periods.

I have met several American qigong pioneers who started practicing in the 1970s. An article in *Qigong & Science* (5, 1995) written by Wang Zhen-Hua says that John Alton went to China in 1987 for help after his doctors told him that even with surgery, there would be no more than a five percent guarantee that his severely injured wrist could recover. John even had to sign a promise that he could not sue his doctor if he removed his wrist protector before a six-month period. During the time he was in China, he learned qigong as well as martial arts from Master Wang Zhen-Hua in Beijing University. Though he also received qigong treatments from Master Wang, John was worried when his qigong teacher threw away his wrist protector. While receiving the treatment, however, his worry evaporated. He felt some pleasant, tickling sensation expanding from his waist to his chest. His injured wrist started moving and his fingers became numb and itchy. A week later, he learned from his teacher how to treat himself. After five months, his wrist recovered.

Ever since then, he and his wife have been practicing and learning more about qigong. They are able to treat and heal themselves now when catching colds. John quit his teaching position in a university after he returned from China and established a qigong and martial arts school named The Three Emperors. He has helped many people recover their health and learn martial arts. For example, a young woman who had chronic heart disease and gynecological problems underwent several operations but who still suffered severe sickness has recovered her health after learning qigong from Mr. Alton. The leg problems of one of his students, Daniel, who also went to Beijing University to learn Chinese, martial arts, and qigong, were healed.

## Translation from Master Ou Wen-Wei's Work

Before I end this book, I would like to offer you a translation as a resource. This article, written by Master Ou Wen-Wei in October 1997 for a lecture titled "Qigong is a Special Sphere of Learning Related to the Material and the Spirit" at a qigong conference, defines qigong from the writer's point of view, I included Ou's story in the section about spirit teachers earlier in this book. His essay won an award for the essay from the International League of Somatic Science in 1995.

> Human spirit (soul/po) is invisible, not an object, not material; it is formed by the life source, thinking ability and the energy from the universe. Channels are the "pipes" of life source (including qi). Acupoints are the cross-joints for all the physiological functions. The fundamental principle of the channels and blood vessels is the same—the channels are "pipes" for qi; and the vessels are the pipes for blood, but the two take different forms. Blood is material, in liquid form and needs to move in solid vessels that are made of fine, firm material. Such vessels enable the blood to flow in specific directions (as do the other parts of circulatory system). Life source is an invisible power, and as other kinds of invisible powers, it can go through space (using space as an energy-carrier), pass through objects (using carriers made of material), and pass power by using the other energies as carriers. The way that life source passes power is like the energy of the territorial gravity of the earth—through space.

*The gravity from the earth can use the earth as the carrier, and also can pass energy through the space. Life source does not need a solid "pipe" to pass its energy. That is the reason why basic anatomy cannot discover or reveal these channels in the human body.*

*For all the physiological functions to work in harmony and in an orderly manner, the life source always chooses the most effective directions to move, thus the channels are formed. Such activity is similar to the magnetic power that always moves to one direction.*

*Qigong is a special, profound field of knowledge that originated in and established during ancient times. Its existence today has revealed that there were super-powered masters in ancient times who have left us a precious science related to the human body. These ancient masters practiced, experienced, developed and have left to us this precious, special knowledge in order to lead and teach us to study the human body. We should really study, carry forward, and develop this field of knowledge objectively.*

*Now there have been several qigong practitioners who "saw", when they were in qigong state, that there were light-nets and some black dots like black sesame seeds inside people's bodies. The light-net and "dots" matched the qi channels and acupoints in the charts of Traditional Chinese Medicine. Interestingly, this psychic power has happened to some of my students. They asked me how to explain this. My definition is: When a person is in a special qigong state, when the condition of body is in correspondence with the life source while it is moving, possibly some parts that turned into light form, then the life source and the light synchronize; the channel-nets and the acupoints appeared. It is not unusual for several qigong practitioners to have psychic power for scanning those lights. The necessary conditions in which those lights are visible to the psychic person is that the other person is in a qigong state, a condition that allows the life source and light to transform. We have not totally learned these natural laws and we should not indulge in seeking to "see" the lights. We should practice and experi-*

*ence such phenomenon cautiously with a tranquil and relaxed mind.*

*Those who have gained much experience through practicing qigong sincerely and through observing and treating patients will gradually and learn deeply that a human being is formed by two parts: a visible, material system and an invisible power system. These two systems can overlap and can join together, and they can also be separate, relatively oppositely. The separation of these two systems creates a better combination.*

*These two systems are related and correspond closely to the visible material and power of the universe. The digestive and breathing systems are the main ways that human beings relate to the outside world. Material that is absorbed through these more physical "canals" is turned into cells and energy. To practice qigong is to allow the energy in the human body to transform in a systematic and effective way. Thus, the energy that is absorbed will change the "material as the main object and energy acts to assist" into its opposite—the energy will become the main force and the material is to assist. Thus, the energy will be involved in the enhancement of life source and immunity, to readjust and normalize, as well as to complement the energy that has been consumed. This is the fundamental reason why practicing qigong can heal and tonify health. That Pan Gu Mystical Qigong can heal patients with conditions such as lupus erythematosus, rheumatoid disease, and dysfunction of adrenal gland, is a proof of the above.*

# Glossary

*Ba Gua.* The ancient theory said handed down by the Emperor-Sage, Fu Xi. The theory defines the relationships between human and nature, and is also used to predict the future.

*Chan.* The Chinese word for the zen practice.

*Cosmic Yang.* Refers to the cosmic qi.

*Dan.* When used as a single word, it is Daoist term. In qigong, it refers to the refined qi.

*Dan Tian.* The two-word term refers to the area where qi is accumulated and forms into da.

*De.* De in Dao De Jing refers to morality.

*Earth Immortals.* A term referring to the qigong masters who achieved the high level state, but have not gotten beyond the earth condition. It is another way to say human immortal.

*Essential Jing.* This is another term that refers to the primary qi.

*Essential Qi.* Also called, "primary qi."

*Extrasensory.* The revealed human potentials such as intuition, scanning ability, etc.

*Five Elements Theory.* A term from qigong theory that is also an integral part of Traditional Chinese Medicine.

*Gold Dan.* A Daoist term referring to the refined and accumulated qi in the dan tian. It also can mean Daoist alchemy.

*Grand Master.* A term referring to the masters who have achieved a certain high level of qigong practice, as well as knowledge about qigong.

*Gua Sha.* A common method of treatment method that many ordinary Chinese people use. A piece of china, ox horn, or clay is used on the skin to treat some illnesses according to the qi acupoints. The treated area of the skin becomes reddish even dark red color after the treatment.

*Heart/mind.* The heart and mind are one word, xin in Chinese language.

*Heavenly Immortals.* Qigong masters who have gained a higher level of achievement beyond the earth level.

*Hua.* A verb that means to change; power that is gained through qigong practice.

*Human Aura.* According to qigong theory, human aura is another form of qi.

*Human Immortals.* This is a different way to refer to earth immortals.

*Human Spirit (soul/po).* As it is used in other cultures, too

*Hun.* Soul

*Hun Po.* A Daoist term for hun and spirit.

*Immortality.* A Daoist term referring to longevity.

*Immortals.* A Daoist term referring to those high-level qigong masters who have gained longevity. The Chinese also use this term to praise an aged person.

*Internal Breathing.* The qigong high-level way of breathing from within.

*Internal Qi.* This term refers to the qi movements that move in the qigong state; also mostly refers to the primary qi.

*Jing (not Ching).* The term used with other words to show a specific meaning. If the word refers to the qigong term, jing, qi and shen, then it means the essence in the qi.

*Ling Hun.* Soul/spirit.

*Live Zi Hour to Harvest the Yao.* A Daoist term referring to the active qi movement from the bottom arousing similar to the sex sensation.

*Longevity Dan.* The accumulated, refined qi in the lower dan tian. It can also refer to the Daoist herbal-mineral alchemy.

*Muddle-Headed State.* This term refers to people who are clueless about life.

*Mudra.* The hand postures in qigong practices.

*Pair Cultivation.* A Daoist term referring to a male and female practicing together.

*Pair-Cultivation Qigong.* The qigong practice and cultivation for the pairs.

*Pi Gu.* To eat qi, a Daoist term.

*Po Strength.* A Chinese term referring to daring, inspiration.

*Positive Energy.* Yang energy, a Daoist term.

*Pure Yang (the Cosmic Yang) State.* A qigong state of a high-level master whose body has gotten rid of all yin energy.

*Qi.* The vital energy in Western terms.

*Qi and Jing.* The Daoist term to referring to the body's energy and the process of qigong.

*Qi Blockages.* Chinese medical term referring to the stagnation of energy.

*Qi Channels.* Qigong and Traditional Chinese Medicine terms refer to the qi that flows through the body.

*Qi Field.* The places affected by qigong practitioners' qi energy at places where they practiced.

*Qi Healer.* Yanling's term to refer to the qi healing process within and during the qigong state.

*Qigong.* Qi energy, the exercise, and the achievements.

*Qigong Doctors.* Qigong healers who have earned good reputations.

*Qigong State.* When the practitioner is in a carefree state and totally relaxed.

*Quan Zhen.* The Daoist term for a Daoist school.

*Real Humans.* The Daoist term referring to immortals.

*Scanning Abilities.* Those who have these abilities can see through self or other people's bodies.

*Semen Jing.* The Chinese medical term for the essence that exists in the semen.

*Seventh Sense.* A Buddhist term referring to the revealed human potential.

*She Li Zi.* The material left by the high-level Buddhist masters after their bodies are cremated.

*Shen.* Spirit.

*Shen Hun.* A term for the mind state.

*Shen Tong.* A term referring to various human extrasensory abilities.

*Shen Xian.* A term for immortals/celestial.

*Shuang Xiu.* A Daoist term for qigong pair-cultivation, study, and practice

*Six Incantations.* A chanting handed down by the Buddha Guanyin.

*Six Sticky Glue Balls.* A metaphor used by the Buddha to refer to emotions.

*Sixth Sense.* A Buddhist term for the extrasensory abilities.

*Soul/Po.* A term for soul.

*Taiji (Tai Chi).* Another term for yin and yang that refers to the natural law.

*Tangled Qi.* Refers to the qi stagnation in the channels.

*Tui Na.* Traditional Chinese Medicine's method of treating the tendons and muscles by using acupoints and qi channels.

*Void State.* This is the same as "the void." The word in Chinese is *xu*.

*Wan.* Empty. A qigong term referring to the wrong way to empty the mind/heart for a long time.

*Xian.* Chinese word for immortal/celestial.

*Xiang (with a falling tone).* Refers the looking of a person, built by life experience and inherited looking.

*Xin.* Chinese word for the heart-mind.

*Xin Zang.* The heart organ.

*Xiu Lian.* A qigong term for practicing, study, and cultivation.

*Xiu Xing (xing read second tone).* A qigong term for cultivating the heart/mind and actions.

*Xiu Xing (Xing read the falling tone).* A term referring to the cultivation of the heart-mind so it returns to its origins.

*Yang Energy.* Positive energy.

*Yang Morality.* Good deeds that are known by people.

*Yang Shen (Yang Spirit).* The high-level refined soul that has cast off yin energy.

*Yang World.* Refers to the world where living people live.

*Yin and Yang.* A Daoist term referring to the natural law; the qi energy that is also used in Chinese medicine.

*Yin Devil.* A term for the world where dead people stay.

*Yin Energy.* Negative energy.

*Yin Morality.* Work on self, doing good deeds, but not caring whether the deeds are known by others.

*Yin Shen.* Invisible spirit; soul that is in refined process.

*Yin-Moral Cultivation.* Refers to people who do good deeds, but not let people know to work on the xin.

*Yuan Shen.* Another term for the primary shen.

*Zhong Qi.* The essential qi.

*Zi Ran.* The Chinese way of referring to nature: naturally there.

# References

ANCIENT

These citations refer to writings that were done in the far past. Some have been re-published by modern organizations and publishing houses. References given here are mostly published in Chinese. Some books are available in full or partial translations, such as the *I Ching* or *Xi You Ji* (*Travel Notes Towards the West*).

*The Ancestors of the Daoist Quan Zhen School*, The White Cloud Monastery

*Ba Gua*, by Emperor Sage Fu Xi

*Bao Pu Zi Nei Pian*, by Ge Hong (283-363 AD), Hui Zhou Publications, Yunnan Province, 1995

*Ben Cao Gangmu Herbal Classic* (updated by Li She-Zhen in the Ming Dynasty)

*Ben Cao Shen Nong Herbal Classic Teachings* (original by the Emperor-Sage Shen Nong)

*The Collections of Ming Dao and Fan Xi*, Authors unknown

*Chun-Yang San Shu*, Immortal Lu Dong-Bin, White Cloud Monastery

*Dao De Jing*, by Lao Zi (Li Den)

*Dao Zang*, (A complete collection of more than 5,000 Daoist books updated in the Song Dynasty)

*The Dragon Gate Xin Fa*, by Qiu Chu-Ji (Yuan Dynasty), Printed by the Mount Hua Daoist Association

*Essential Prescriptions Worth a Thousand Gold Tablets*, by Sun Si-Miao (Tang Dynasty)

*General Treatise on the Etiology and Symptomology*, by Chao Yuan-Fang (550-630 AD)

*Guan Zi*, by Guan Zi, The People's Health Publications, 1954

*The Guidance of Cultivation Through Da Dan*, Author unknown

*Han Shu* (Chapter of *Yi Wen Zhi* written in Han Dynasty), The Chinese Classic Medical Book Publications, Beijing, 1954

*How to Predict the Future*, by Zhu Ge-Liang (188-263 BC), Edited by Shao Kang-Jie (960-1217 AD) Lao Gu Publication, Taiwan, 1979

*I Ching*, Author unknown

*The Immortal Classic*, by Lu Dong-Bin (Tang Dynasty), updated by the White Cloud Monastery

*Immortal Qiu's Trip to the West*, by Li Zhi-Chang

*Jin Ping Mei* (*The Plum In a Gold Vase*), by Xiao Xiao-Sheng (a pen name, Ming Dynasty)

*Lei Jing*, by Zhang Jie-Bin (Ming Dynasty), The People's Health Publications, 1964

*Ling Shu Classic*, Author unknown (about 475-221 BC)

*My Family's Teaching—Establish Own Fate*, by Yuan Liao-Fan (Ming Dynasty), White Cloud Monastery

*Notes on a Geographical Expedition*, by Xu Xia-Ke (Ming Dynasty)

*Shan Hai Jing*, Author unknown (about 3,000 years ago)

*TCM and the I Ching*, by Zhang Jie-Bin (Ming dynasty) Beijing Xue Yuan Publication, 1993

*The Variorum of the Herbal Classic*, by Tao Hong-Jing (Tang Dynasty)

*Xi You Ji (Travel Notes Towards the West)* , by Wu Chen-En (Ming Dynasty)

*Xuan Ji Direct Definition*, by Immortal Zhang San-Feng

*The Yellow Emperor Essential Internal (Nei) Jing*, Author unknown (written about 3,000 years ago)

*Yin Fu Jing*, Author unknown (prior to Han Dynasty)

*Yoga Ancestors' Teachings* (Buddhist Miluo's lectures), Translated by Master Monk Xuan Zhuang (Tang Dynasty), Xinfeng Publications, Taiwan

*Zhou Yi Tsan Tong Qi*, by Immortal Wei Bo-Yang (Han Dynasty)

*Zun Sheng*, by Gao Lian (Ming Dynasty)

## CONTEMPORARY PUBLICATIONS

These references were written or compiled in recent times. Only some are available in English.

*Ancient Well-Known Physicians Define Zhou I Ching*, Edited by He Shao-Chu, The Chinese TCM and Science Publication Co., 1991

*Answers to 120 Questions about Tibetan Buddhism*, by Rinpoche Luosangtudanqongpai, Sichuan Minzu Publications, 2000

*The Chinese Secretly Handed Down Precious Classic*, by Daoist Physician Zhu Heh-Ting, Hong Kong Asian Arts Publications, 1994

*The Chinese Treasure of Secret Qian Dao*, by Liu Heh-Ting, Hong Kong Asian Arts Publications, 1994

*The Daoist Religion and Preserving Faith*, by Daoist Master Yun Dunzi, The Chinese National Daoist Association, 1969

*The Daoist Religion and Preserving Health and Longevity*, by Chen Ying-Ning, Hua Wen Publications, Beijing, www.hwcbs.com

*The Daoist School of Gui Yuan*, by Zhen Yangzi, Da Lian City Publications, Shen Yang Province, 1994

*The Definition of Dao De Jing*, by Zhan Yangzi, Da Lian Publications, 1994

*The Definition of the Zhou Yi*, by Gao Hen, Zhong Hua Book Publications, 1984

*Fragrant and Wisdom Qigong*, by Tian Rui-Sheng, Beijing Physical Education College, 1992

*Guide to Immortality*, by Daoist and TCM Dr. Hu Hai-Ya, The Chinese Classic Medical Publications, Beijing, 1998

*Herbal Food for Longevity and Vitality*, compiled by Yanling Lee Johnson, Manuscript to be published

*Immortality and Longevity*, by Chen Ying-Ning, Chinese National Daoist Association

*Introduction to the Daoist Holistic Zhen School*, Compiled and published by the White Cloud Monastery, 1997

*Leng Jia Buddhist Classic* (Buddha's teachings collected by his students), Defined by Master Nan Huai-Jin

*The Longevity Gong*, by Master Zhu Hui, Zheijang Publications, 1997

*Modern Qigongology*, by Dr. Feng Li-Da, Economic Science Publications, Beijing, 1994

*Notes on the I Ching*, by Nan Huai-Jin, The World Languages Publication, 1989

*Qi, The Treasure and Power of Your Body*, by Yanling Lee Johnson, Qigong Association of America, 1996

*Qigong & Science* (magazine published in China)

*Qigong in Modern Science*, by Dr. Feng Li-Da, Economic Science Publications, Beijing, 1999

*Shaolin Kungfu Photo Book*, Editorial Committee of Shao Lin Monastery, 1994

*Supplementary Definitions of the I Ching*, The World Languages Publication, 1991

*Ten Thousands of No Doings*, Edited by Fan Xian-Qing, The Farm Publication, He Fei Shandong Province, 1991

*The Thirty-Four Ancient Well-Known Experts' Definitions of Zhou Yi San Tong Qi*, Hua Xia Publications, 1993)

*To Study the I Ching*, by Chen Ming-Hong, Zhi Shang Publications, Taiwan, 1954

*Wei Mo Essential House*, by Yuan Huan-Xian, Lao Gu Publications, Taiwan

*A Woman's Qigong Guide*, by Yanling Lee Johnson, YMAA Publication Center, Boston, 2001

*The Yuan Jue Buddhist Classic*, Defined by Nan Huai-Jin, Lao Gu Publications, Taiwan

*Zhou I Ching*, Defined by Li Chiang, The Culture of Religion Publications

OTHER PUBLICATIONS IN CHINESE THAT INCLUDE DESCRIPTIONS OF MODERN EXPERIMENTS

*The 3.1.2 Channels Exercises for Seniors*, Edited by Zhu Zong-Xiang, Puzi Science Publications, 1994

*Chinese Medical Qigong*, Edited by Song Tian-Bin and Liu Yuan-Liang, The People's Health Publications, 1994

*Clinical Medical Qigong*, by Gao Wei-Bin, Cheng Wei-Ping, and Hu Jie, Chinese Medical Science and Technical Publications, 1989

*Comprehensive Guide to Medical Qigong*, by Zhang Xia and Tian Jin, Chinese Science and Technical Publications, 1990

*Detecting Diseases by Checking Palms*, by Wang Chen-Xia, Gansu Minorities
    Publications, 1993

*Illustrations of Detecting Diseases by Checking Palms*, by Wang Da-You,
    Beijing Science and Technical Publications, 1995

*Jiao Guo-Rui Qigong in Preserving Health*, by Jiao Gao-Rui, Huaxia
    Publications, 1955

*MCM Medical Qigong*, Edited by Xue Li-Gong *et al.*, Heilongjiang Science
    and Technical Publications, 1989.

*The Newest Treatments for Pain Caused by Cancer*, by Zheng Yu-Ling,
    Chinese Traditional Medicine Publications, 1993

*The Qigong Daoyin*, by Tao Pin-Fu and Yao Shan-Yu, Chinese Science
    and Technical Publications, 1991

*Qigong Explorations of the Secrets*, by Tao Bin-Fu, Chinese Science and
    Technical Publications, 1991

*Qigong in Preserving Lives*, by the Association of Book Collections for
    Preserving Lives, Jiangsu Provincial Science and Technology
    Publications, 1992

*Qigong in Treating Cancer*, by Wang Yin, Shanxi Provincial Science and
    Technical Publications, 1994

*The Scientific Foundation of Qigong*, by Xie Huan-Zhang, The Culture of
    Preserving Health Publications, 1991

*TCM Breathing Studies*, by Yan Li, , Bejing Science and Technical
    Publications, 1995

*TCM in Detecting Diseases*, by Yang Li, Bejing Science and Technical
    Publications, 1988

*World Qigong* (a journal originally edited by Master Xu Xian-Tang and
    published by The World Medical Qigong Association, now
    discontinued)

RECOMMENDED RESOURCES

International Yan Xin Qigong Association 614 374-0023 (fax).

The Qigong Association Of America, www.qi.org, or call 541 745-6310
    (includes information about Grand Master Wang Zi-Sheng)

ZY Qigong Association, Grand Master Xu Ming-Tang's website,
    www.qigong.ru and email qigong@w-link.net.

*The Travels of Marco Polo (Il milione)*, by Marco Polo

Books by Dr. Yang Jwing-Ming published by the YMAA Publication
    Center

*Qigong—the Energy for Life*, by James MacRichie, Collins, London, 2002

*An Open Heart*, Dalai Lama and Nicholas Vreeland, Little Brown &
    Company, New York, 2001

*The Empty Vessel* (magazine published by The Abode of the Eternal Tao)

*The Dragon Mouth* (the British Daoist magazine)

*Shaolin Kungfu* (magazine published by Pacific Rim Publishing)

# Index

acupuncture 26
adenocarcinoma 149-151
Alton, John 164-167
animals 40
astronomy 62
athletes 156-157
aura 93
Avalokitesvara 132
Ba Gua 22
Bao Puzi 74, 117
bedroom skills 107, 116, 118, 120
blood circulation 160-161
blood pressure 154-155
boat (bodily form) 8
Boddhidharma 6
Bodhisattva 113, 132
bodies, moving other peoples 85-87
bone disease 82
brain 67, 161-162
Buddha 12
Buddha levels 46
Buddhism 4, 47
Buddhist nuns 47, 99-100
cancer 149, 151-152
carcinoma 149-151, 150-152
celestials 15, 44, 46
chan 6, 11
chanting 138
Chen Mu 6
Chen Ying-Ning 20, 23, 109
Chen Ying-Zi 113-114
Cheng Hui-Xian 86-87
children 9, 90-91, 148-149
Chinese mythology 4
cholesterol 159-160
clinical investigations 140-141
colors 4
Confucianism 100
cultivation 69, 71, 74, 125
Da Ming Incantation 132
Da Mo 6
Dao 18, 22
Dao De Jing 20, 23
Dao Hong-Jing 117
Daoism 4, 20, 111
Daoist schools 108, 109
deities 4
Dematis, Russel 94
Deng Xiao-Ping xii
Ding Hou-Di 153-154
Dong Hua 50

Dragon Gate 110, 112-113
Dragon of Fire 59
drowsiness 128
drug 32
Eight Immortals 49
electromagnetic waves 33
Emperor-Sage Yao 116-117
extrasensory abilities 5, 68, 69
eye exercises 146-147
Fang Ting-Yu 29
female practitioner 102
Feng Li-Da 149-151, 150-152, 163-165
fire element 66
Five Element Theory 83, 130-131
funeral 13
gallstones 155-156
Gao Wen-Ju 57
Genghis Khan 56
ghost immortals 45
Gu Han-Sen 164-165
Guan Yin 113, 132
Guan Zi 5
Gui Xian 45
Guo Lin vii
Guo Lin Qigong viii
Hai Deng 49
Han Xiang-Zi 52
healing 8, 29, 146-147
heart disease 157-159
heart-mind 66
heaven 14
heavenly immortals 46
Heh Bin-Hui 151-152
Heh Xian-Gu 53
hell 14
herbs 30
Holistic Zhen Daoism 60
Hu Hai-Ya 36-37, 111
Hu Song-Chang 146
hua 66
Hua Yang 50
human aura 93
human immortals 45
hun po 16
I Ching 20, 21, 22
ill thoughts 126
immortality 36, 99-100, 107
incantations 129-130
inner being 70
intuition 67, 69
invisible spirit 42

Jiang Chang-Wen x
jing 5, 104
Ju-Qing Qian 149-151
kidneys 121, 140-141
Kun Dao 47
Lan Tsai-Heh 52
Li Shen-Ping 34
Li Si-Chen 157-159
Li Tie-Guai 51
Li Yu-Lin 110-111
Li Zhi-Chang 56
Li Hong-Zhi 69
lights 139
Liu Zhu-Qiang 156-157
live zi hour 105-106
liver 155-156
Lock the Gold Cabinet In the Dream
    Qigong 122-123
longevity 120-121, 131
Lu Dong-Bin 19, 39-41, 54, 65
Lu Zi-Yin 144
Lu Zu-Yin 34
Ma Wang Dui Guide Hypnotize Qigong
    80
Ma Wang Dui Tomb 79, 87-89, 116-117,
    118
Mai Yan-Qiong 82
Majilaya 48
mammary gland hyperplasia 148-149
Marco Polo 12
Master Situ Qi vii
meditation 105, 115, 127-128, 133
melatonin 143
Ming-Lian 48
moral cultivation 71
mummies 95
muscles 153-154
Nan Huai-Jin 14, 74, 106, 111
nao 67
negative energy 70, 126
numbers 62
Ou Wen-Wei 40, 165-168
oxygen consumption 145
pair cultivation 109-110
Pan Gu 4
Panchans 96
Peng Zu 4, 117
physical body 62
pi gu 87-89, 151-152
pi qi 133
pineal gland 143
Po 16
Potidarmo 6
practice 7, 69, 74
practice, self-effort 7, 8
prevention 32

primary qi 37-38, 105-106
primary spirit 43
pulse 159-160
qi 35, 62, 93, 104
qi channels 11, 64
qi energy 27, 33-34, 144
qi engine 124
qi fields 82
qi healing 31
qi movement 115
Qian Dao 47
Qian Long 57
qigong 2, 3, 7, 69
Qigong & Science ix
qigong masters, ancient 4, 39, 95-96
qigong masters, modern x, xii, 163-165
qigong practice 2, 11, 64, 74, 87-89, 105-
    106, 124, 127
qigong practitioners, female 102
qigong research institutes x
qigong skills 78
qigong theory 21, 29, 140
qigong, and acupuncture 26
qigong, modern developments vii
qigong, Tibetan 12
Qiu 55-56
Qiu Chu-Ji 76, 112-113
quan zhen 111-112
Quan Zhen School 108, 112
rainbow lights 94-95
reincarnation 13
relaxation 124-125
remains 46
Rinpoche Luosangtudanpai 13, 69
Roman spectrum 34
Rotating Qigong 91-92
saliva 145
scanning 163-164
Seed of Buddha 11
self-cultivation 137
self-effort 18, 74
senile dementia 138
seniors 145-146
senses 72-73
seven-day cycle 64
sex 103-104
sex changes 113
sexual arousal 105, 115
sexual relationship 99
Shaolin monks 79
she li zi 46, 95
Shen 15, 104, 126
Shen Nong 4
Shen Tong 38-39, 67, 69
Shi Hong Qing 89-91
side effects 32

Six Exhaling Sounds Exercise 129
Six Incantations 132
six sticky glue balls 72
Soaring Crane Qigong viii
sons 100
soul 1, 8, 9, 11, 13, 65, 67
sounds 130, 138
Southern Daoist School 109-110
space simulation 91-92
spirit 1, 16, 65
spirit masters 43
stress 145
Sun Si-Miao 117, 120
Tai Chi Wu Xing Gong 151-152
taiji 22, 60
Tang Mei-Tsi 146
teacher 125, 127
temperature 160-161
tendons 153-154
terminally ill patients 151-152
third eye 163-164
Thirteen Movements 60
thought transmittance 81-82
Tian 3
Tian Rei-Shen 94
tian xian 44, 46
Tibetan Buddhism 47
Tibetan Mi Zong 47
timing 27, 133
Tong Zun-Jie 79
Traditional Chinese Medicine 26, 30, 31, 140
triglyceride 159-160
trigram symbol 22
Tsao Guo-Jiu 51
Tsongkhapa 109
tumors 150-152
Vermanns, Erice Yao 41
vessels 62-63
vitality 64
void state 105, 136
Wang Chang-Yin 155-156
Wang Chong-Yang 112
Wang You-Cheng 81
Wang Zhen-Hua 164-167
Wang Zi-Shen 12, 132
water 138
Wei Bo-Yang 5
Wen Si-Xian 88-90
Western medicine 29
Wild Goose Qigong viii
women, status of 99
Wu Chen-En 76
Wu Dang style 60
Wu Ji 96-97
Wu Jiang 41

Wu Long-Chang 154-155
Wu Meng 6
Wu Ze-Tian 50, 54, 101
xian 15, 36-37
Xian Jing 121-122
xin 66, 67, 126
xing 103-104
Xu Mi 39-41
Xu Ming-Tang 33, 94, 145
Xu Xia-Ke 98
Xu Xun 5
Xuan Zhen Guan 110-111
Xuan Zong 51, 101
Yan Xin 3, 34, 83, 84-85, 93-94, 144
yang 44
Yang morality 71
yang qi 93
Yang Shen 16, 41, 43
yang spirits 46, 72
Yang Xi 39-41
Yang Yu-Huan 101
yao 3, 105-106, 121-122
Yellow Emperor 4, 117
Yi Zhi Chan Gong 153-154
yin 11
yin and yang theory 119-120
yin devil 70
yin moral belief 11
yin morality 71
Yin Shen 16, 41, 42
yin world 14
Yixitsojie 48
Yong-Tai 48
Yu Zhen 51
Yu Zhu-Tian 156-157
Yuan Huang 23
Yuan Shen 43
Yun Duanzi 36-38, 44
Yun Gu 24
Zhang Guo-Lao 50
Zhang Jian-Zhou 163-165
Zhang Rong-Tang 91-92
Zhang San-Feng 38, 43, 57-59
Zhang Zhen-Huan vii, xi
Zhang Zi-Yang 110-111
Zhao Fei-Yan 101
zhen ren 36-37, 41, 44
Zhen Yangzi 16
Zhong Li-Quan 50, 54
Zhong Yuan Qigong 94
Zhu Chang-Ya 18
Zhu Heh-Ting 116, 120-121
Zhuang Zi 111-112

# BOOKS FROM YMAA PUBLICATION CENTER

| | |
|---|---|
| B041/868 | 101 Reflections on Tai Chi Chuan |
| B031/582 | 108 Insights into Tai Chi Chuan—A String of Pearls |
| B046/906 | 6 Healing Movements—Qigong for Health, Strength, & Longevity |
| B045/833 | A Woman's Qigong Guide—Empowerment through Movement, Diet, and Herbs |
| B009/041 | Analysis of Shaolin Chin Na—Instructor's Manual for all Martial Styles |
| B004R/671 | Ancient Chinese Weapons—A Martial Artist's Guide |
| B015R/426 | Arthritis—The Chinese Way of Healing and Prevention (formerly Qigong for Arthritis) |
| B030/515 | Back Pain—Chinese Qigong for Healing and Prevention |
| B020/300 | Baguazhang—Emei Baguazhang |
| B043/922 | Cardio Kickboxing Elite—For Sport, for Fitness, for Self-Defense |
| B028/493 | Chinese Fast Wrestling for Fighting—The Art of San Shou Kuai Jiao |
| B016/254 | Chinese Qigong Massage—General Massage |
| B057/043 | Chinese Tui Na Massage—The Essential Guide to Treating Injuries, Improving Health, & Balancing Qi |
| B038/809 | Complete CardioKickboxing—A Safe & Effective Approach to High Performance Living |
| B021/36x | Comprehensive Applications of Shaolin Chin Na—The Practical Defense of Chinese Seizing Arts for All Styles |
| B010R/523 | Eight Simple Qigong Exercises for Health—The Eight Pieces of Brocade |
| B025/353 | The Essence of Shaolin White Crane—Martial Power and Qigong |
| B014R/639 | The Essence of Taiji Qigong—The Internal Foundation of Taijiquan (formerly Tai Chi Chi Kung) |
| B062/213 | The Fighting Arts—Their Evolution from Secret Societies to Modern Times |
| B017R/345 | How to Defend Yourself—Effective & Practical Martial Arts Strategies |
| B056/108 | Inside Tai Chi—Hints, Tips, Training, & Process for Students & Teachers |
| B033/655 | The Martial Arts Athlete—Mental and Physical Conditioning for Peak Performance |
| B042/876 | Mind/Body Fitness |
| B061/183 | Mugai Ryu—The Classical Samurai Art of Drawing the Sword |
| B006R/85x | Northern Shaolin Sword—Forms, Techniques, and Applications |
| B044/914 | Okinawa's Complete Karate System—Isshin-Ryu |
| B037/760 | Power Body—Injury Prevention, Rehabilitation, and Sports Performance Enhancement |
| B050/99x | Principles of Traditional Chinese Medicine—The Essential Guide to Understanding the Human Body |
| B012R/841 | Qigong—The Secret of Youth |
| B005R/574 | Qigong for Health and Martial Arts—Exercises and Meditation (formerly Chi Kung—Health & Martial Arts) |
| B058/116 | Qigong for Living—A Practical Guide for Improving Your Health with Qi from Modern China |
| B040/701 | Qigong for Treating Common Ailments—The Essential Guide to Self-Healing |
| B011R/507 | The Root of Chinese Qigong—Secrets for Health, Longevity, & Enlightenment |
| B055/884 | Shihan-Te—The Bunkai of Kata |
| B049/930 | Taekwondo—Ancient Wisdom for the Modern Warrior |
| B059/221 | Taekwondo—Spirit & Practice |
| B032/647 | The Tai Chi Book—Refining and Enjoying a Lifetime of Practice |
| B019R/337 | Tai Chi Chuan—24 & 48 Postures with Martial Applications (formerly Simplified Tai Chi Chuan) |
| B008R/442 | Tai Chi Chuan Martial Applications—Advanced Yang Style (formerly Advanced Yang Style Tai Chi Chuan, v.2) |
| B035/71x | Tai Chi Secrets of the Ancient Masters—Selected Readings with Commentary |
| B047/981 | Tai Chi Secrets of the W«u & Li Styles—Chinese Classics, Translations, Commentary |
| B054/175 | Tai Chi Secrets of the Wu Styles—Chinese Classics, Translations, Commentary |
| B048/094 | Tai Chi Secrets of the Yang Style—Chinese Classics, Translations, Commentary |
| B007R/434 | Tai Chi Theory & Martial Power—Advanced Yang Style (formerly Advanced Yang Style Tai Chi Chuan, v.1) |
| B060/23x | Tai Chi Walking—A Low-Impact Path to Better Health |
| B022/378 | Taiji Chin Na—The Seizing Art of Taijiquan |
| B036/744 | Taiji Sword, Classical Yang Style—The Complete Form, Qigong, and Applications |
| B034/68x | Taijiquan, Classical Yang Style—The Complete Form and Qigong |
| B046/892 | Traditional Chinese Health Secrets—The Essential Guide to Harmonious Living |
| B039/787 | Wild Goose Qigong—Natural Movement for Healthy Living |
| B027/361 | Wisdom's Way—101 Tales of Chinese Wit |
| B013R/416 | Xingyiquan—Theory, Applications, Fighting Tactics, & Spirit |

## YMAA PUBLICATION CENTER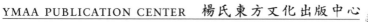

4354 Washington Street Roslindale, MA 02131
1-800-669-8892 • ymaa@aol.com • www.ymaa.com

# home book of SMOKE-COOKING
## Meat, Fish & Game